I0019503

JOURNAL OF GREEN ENGINEERING

Aims and Scopes
Journal of Green Engineering will publish original, high quality, peer-reviewed research papers and review articles dealing with environmentally safe engineering including their systems. Paper submission is solicited on:

- Theoretical and numerical modeling of environmentally safe electrical engineering devices and systems.
- Simulation of performance of innovative energy supply systems including renewable energy systems, as well as energy harvesting systems.
- Modeling and optimization of human environmentally conscientiousness environment (especially related to electromagnetics and acoustics).
- Modeling and optimization of applications of engineering sciences and technology to medicine and biology.
- Advances in modeling including optimization, product modeling, fault detection and diagnostics, inverse models.
- Advances in software and systems interoperability, validation and calibration techniques. Simulation tools for sustainable environment (especially electromagnetic, and acoustic).
- Experiences on teaching environmentally safe engineering (including applications of engineering sciences and technology to medicine and biology).

All these topics may be addressed from a global scale to a microscopic scale, and for different phases during the life cycle.

JOURNAL OF GREEN ENGINEERING

Volume 2   No. 1   October 2011

Published, sold and distributed by:
River Publishers
P.O. Box 1657
Algade 42
9000 Aalborg
Denmark

Tel.: +45369953197
www.riverpublishers.com

Journal of Green Engineering is published four times a year.
Publication programme, 2011–2012: Volume 2 (4 issues)

ISSN 1904-4720

Greening of Video Streaming to Mobile Devices by Pervasive Wireless CDN

Dragan Boscovic[1], Faramak Vakil[1], Staniša Dautović[2]
and Milenko Tošić[3]

[1]*Motorola Mobility, 600 US Highway 45, Libertyville, IL 60048, USA;*
e-mail: dragan.boscovic@motorola.com, faramak.vakil@motorola.com
[2]*Faculty of Technical Sciences, UNS, Trg Dositeja Obradovica 6, 21000 Novi Sad,*
Serbia; e-mail: dautovic@uns.ac.rs
[3]*La Citadelle Inzenjering, Narodnog Fronta 35, 21000 Novi Sad, Serbia;*
e-mail: milenko.tosic@lacitadelleing.com

Received 29 July 2011; Accepted: 5 September 2011

Abstract

Content Delivery Networks (CDNs) play an important role in today's video distribution solutions. While the need for efficient content delivery is well understood, the energy consumption of various video CDN topologies deserves extra attention since energy considerations are increasingly becoming a key performance factor for system designers and operators. This paper investigates the energy efficiency aspect of a special class of video CDN system, namely pervasive wireless CDN based on wireless mesh network implementation. We start by analyzing and defining the energy efficiency of a generic video CDN system. Then we introduce mathematical analysis and simulation model description for wireless CDNs exploring the idea of content placement among wireless access points which serve as local video servers. Computer simulation analysis, based on mixed integer linear programming model, is used to derive "optimal" content placement and caching strategies while minimizing the energy consumption subject to a constraint in terms of the storage size at each mesh router. The objective function of the mathematical model captures the desire to optimize multiple performance

Journal of Green Engineering, Vol. 2, 1–27.

factors. In this particular case we are focusing on the QoS/latency time and power consumption. The results demonstrate trade-off dependency between QoS and power consumption. In summary, the paper offers additional insight into the content diffusion strategies as related to a pervasive wireless CDN, and implications of the placement strategies relative to its energy efficiency.

Keywords: Wireless Mesh Network (WMN), energy efficiency, CDN, video streaming, caching, average delivery tree length.

1 Introduction

Distribution of video over high-speed networks plays important role in many multimedia applications, such as video-on-demand, IPTV, and distance learning. Since video application needs real-time transmission and tight quality of service, the Content Delivery Network is usually used in order to meet these requirements. Through the edge servers deployed close to the end users, the service providers address performance requirements in terms of the access delay and solution scalability.

Nowadays, the operator overlays a content delivery network on top of its existing transport, control, and management infrastructure in order to offer on-demand and time shifted video streaming services to its users. In its generic architecture, a CDN comprises a central library at the original, and several replica server clusters residing at the edge of the network that are mutually interlinked and communicate with each other. Such an overlay network is further connected to users' appliances and devices (e.g. STBs, smart-phones, etc.) through the operator's access (e.g., CATV, wireless, etc.) networks. The original server is the main repository of the CDN where all contents originally reside in and come from its database. Each of the replica servers usually acts both as a content server as well as a cache server hosting a subset of the contents of the original server in its database. The CDN management system places, moves, and replaces the content files across each replica server in accordance to its replica placement and en-route caching algorithms in order to ensure the "optimal" performance and operation of the CDN in the face of the dynamic demand of its user population. A simplified Video CDN topology is shown in Figure 1.

The edge servers are geographically distributed and are generally used to stream video to its local end users. The content replication and propagation to the edge servers is governed by carefully designed policies, which usually calculate content popularity in terms of temporal and spatial viewing patterns.

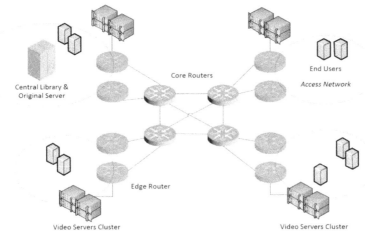

Figure 1 A generic distributed CDN topology.

Relative to serving all the requested content from the original servers, this decentralized approach brings significant advantages in terms of access time and scalability performance. These benefits will normally come at the cost of using more servers and needing more complex management algorithms to support the predictive content replication, updates and distribution. Note that an actual implementation of a given video CDN solution may be more complex than that shown, for example, the video servers can be organized in a multi-tier hierarchy.

When a user's request for content traverses a replica server, it intercepts and examines the message to determine whether it has the requested content. If so, it will serve the request as long as it is not overloaded. Otherwise, it forwards the request to origin server or another replica server for service. Hence, in the current paradigm, a single server, either the origin or a replica/cache server, streams all chunks of the content to the user.

Recently the energy consumption of IT and networking infrastructure has attracted significant attention since the number of server farms is growing and it is estimated that ICT already accounts for $>10\%$ of the overall energy consumption in developed countries. Energy consumption is thus considered as an important factor of IT and Communication system design [1].

In recent publications [2, 3] interdependency between video CDNs topology and energy efficiency has been established. Definition of energy efficiency for a video CDN system has been established by Boscovic et al. [2], while comparison of energy efficiencies between a centralized video delivery system and a distributed CDN system has been provided in [3]. This paper goes one step further and examines diffusive content placement policy in a pervasive mobile mesh CDN wherein each mesh router can serve as a replica/cache server. After describing the need and merits of wireless Mesh CDN, in Sections 3 and 4 we are laying out mathematical framework for understanding principles behind energy consumption considerations for video CDNs, with a special emphasis on wireless CDN topology. Section 4 goes one step further to offer ideas on possible improvements in terms of content replication and management that are likely to yield better energy performance. These recommendations have been validated by means of carefully devised computer simulations and results will be presented in Section 4.

2 Pervasive Wireless Video CDN

As smart-phone penetration and the volume of video traffic on mobile networks increases, Content Delivery Networks (CDNs) are becoming important factor in the mobile landscape. CDNs are important for both operators and content providers as they seek to strengthen their presence in the mobile market.

It is fair to say that market for mobile CDN services has not hit its stride yet; nevertheless it will be a key growth area in the scenarios where offered services are based on delivering the video content. Mobile video traffic is poised to increase exponentially as usage of high-end mobile devices like smart-phones and tablets ramps up. According to Yankee Group's Global Mobile Forecast [4] fewer than 600 million smart-phones will be in use in 2010, but that number will more than double in 2014 to nearly 1.4 billion elevating mobile video to 66% of the total mobile data traffic.

The end-user experience is important to content providers because it will determine how often their servers are hit by the user requests. If content on a given CDN can be viewed easily and with low latency, then user experience and service rating goes up. These issues have been around a while for fixed networks, but now they are becoming just as important for mobile.

The constraints and impairments associated with wireless video delivery are significantly more severe than those associated with wire line. Three of the primary issues that must be dealt with for wireless video distribution are:

- Mobile Device CPU, screen and battery limitations: Mobile devices, particularly those with smaller form factors, utilize processors with lower capability than those in tablets. In addition, the set of display sizes and resolutions can vary greatly. For these reasons it is critical that the video assets be transcoded into formats and "gear sets" that ensure both good quality and efficient use of resources for transmission and decoding. Mobile devices are typically multi-use communication devices on which customers depend for multi-day availability between charges and the battery current drain required for video delivery must be minimized.

- Wireless channel throughput impairments and constraints: Due to the lower available bandwidth and typically smaller displays on mobile devices, the "gear sets" selected for wireless are very different than those for wire line. For example, a mobile device with a 640 × 480 display can work with video bitrates anywhere between 0.16 and 1.0 Mbps, as opposed to 2.5Mbps required by a 1280 × 720 display.

- Diverse wireless Radio Access Network (RAN) types (e.g. Wi-Fi, LTE, WiMAX, etc.): Video delivery solutions should be RAN agnostic. Should the client side control the requested video bit rate, differences in RAN performance can be automatically accommodated as long as there are enough "gears" provided to span the required range.

A pervasive wireless mesh CDN will be an embedded part of the CDN operator's network, control and management infrastructure. Its mesh routers are equipped with required intelligence and storage so it can serve as a dispersed cache/replica server system within and under the control of the operator's CDN management system. At its most basic level, the concept of pervasive wireless CDNs offers simple node caching to help with traffic distribution across the network elements and deliver content with low latency and high user experience. This is very much in line with the vision outlined in [5] by which processing resources are attached to memory resources in order to cut down on the need for data transportation and consequently reduce energy use. This is in contrast to today's computational paradigm in which the microprocessor is in the centre of the computing universe, and information is moved back and forth at heavy energy cost. In addition to the traffic balancing benefits the mobile CDNs hold promise for value add services that can be interpreted as the "special sauce" needed by mobile operators to differentiate their video offerings. Examples of these value added services may include:

- *Device profiling*: With device detection capabilities the mobile CDN is able to detect the screen size/resolution and other graphics performance of the attached device and decide on the best possible delivery mechanisms to maximize the viewing experience.

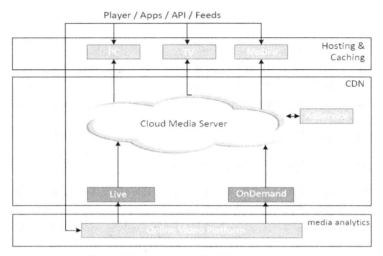

Figure 2 Future composite CDN ecosystem.

- *Scalability*: Content providers do not want to keep changing the way their content is accessed each time a new device debuts. Mobile CDN scalability enables the URL on content provider sites to remain unchanged, even as the content is conditioned (dynamically or statically) and delivery is changed to accommodate a new device.
- *Analytics*: As mobile video delivery takes off, data about who is accessing what content becomes more valuable. Mobile CDNs can report this data back to whatever analytics system the carrier uses.

Services shown in Figure 2 can be all provided within a single CDN or through aggregation. For example, a CDN provider can support media adaptation and conditioning for smart phones and tablets on its own platform, and then for broader device support, it partners with mobile providers that built out their applications over the CDN's operator infrastructure. These mobile providers handle the other value added services, like the handset profiling and on-the-fly content encoding listed above.

3 Energy Efficiency of the Video CDN

We define energy efficiency of a video delivery solution as the amount of concurrent video streams served at requested quality divided by the total energy used for the streaming transaction:

$$\text{efficiency}_{\text{CDN}} = \frac{N_{\text{streams}}}{E_{\text{total}}} \tag{1}$$

This is a relatively broad definition as used in [2], and here focus is not on defining actual measurement metrics or reference workloads. Instead, we would factorize the above efficiency definition into a number of constituting components that can be independently measured and optimized within related engineering disciplines in order to help us identify opportunities for energy saving. As shown in Figure 1, a video CDN comprises a web of data centres and/or servers. The efficiency of each CDN video server site, whether it is a dedicated data centre or a simple server, can be modelled by the following equation:

$$\text{efficiency}_{\text{DC}} = \frac{N_{\text{streams}_{\text{DC}}}}{E_{\text{total}_{\text{DC}}}} = \frac{1}{\text{PUE}} \times \frac{1}{\text{SPUE}} \times \frac{N_{\text{streams}_{\text{DC}}}}{E_{\text{streamings\&storage}_{\text{DC}}}} \tag{2}$$

The above definition is conformant with the Green Grids Data Centre Performance Efficiency (DCPE) definition as given in [6]. The first term in equation (2) relates to the power usage effectiveness (PUE), and reflects energy efficiency of the building infrastructure hosting the CDN servers. It is expressed as the ratio between total power brought to the building, and the power consumed by the actual computing equipment (servers, storage, networking equipment, etc.). The second factor in equation (2) accounts for inefficiencies within the IT equipment itself. Substantial amounts of power may be lost in the servers and network storage power supplies, voltage regulator modules (VRMs), and cooling fans and the SPUE factor reflects these electrical losses. It is defined as the ratio of total server input power and the useful power, where useful power is qualified as being the power consumed by the electronic components directly involved in the video streaming tasks. The PUE and SPUE factors are agnostic to the nature of the service and/or processing load and this paper will not address any specific saving measures as related to them.

    The third term of (2) accounts for energy used, in the case of video CDNs, to support specific number of concurrent video streams. Ultimately, in the context of video CDNs we would like to measure the amount of concurrent video streams delivered by the network from the perspective of the energy invested in the related computational tasks across all the servers/data centres constituting a given CDN.

The total energy consumed by a distributed CDN system should also account for the energy consumed by the interconnecting network. In order to transition from energy efficiency of a self contained data centre to a distributed CDN constellation we invoke efficiency analysis of parallel computing [7]:

$$\text{efficiency}_{\text{CDN}} = \frac{N_{\text{streams}_{\text{CDN}}}}{E_{\text{total}_{\text{CDN}}}} = \left[\frac{\alpha}{\beta} + (1 - \alpha)\right] \times \text{efficiency}_{\text{DC}} \qquad (3)$$

As a CDN is an assembly of mutually interconnected data centres and/or servers, the overall efficiency has to factor for efficiency of each CDN geographical edge server/data centre. Equally it has capacity to account for energy efficiency of the CDN topology, the energy toll of the interconnecting network and efficiency of the content management algorithms. These various energy considerations are modelled by parameters α and β in equation (3). The factor β defines the increase ratio in terms of processing and storage resources deployed in a CDN overlay network relative to the reference VoD data centre. For the sake of simplicity, we assume extra IT resources linearly increase energy consumption within a given video CDN network:

$$E_{\text{total}_{\text{CDN}}} = \beta \times E_{\text{total}_{\text{DC}}} \qquad (4)$$

Parameter α represents the extent to which these additional resources contribute to servicing additional video streams. The border case for $\alpha = 0$ signifies a design in which all additional resources are used to increase the number of serviced video streams; in contrast the design for which $\alpha = 1$ corresponds to the case where all additional resources in a given CDN constellation are used for other purposes (e.g. to improve content access time) and do not contribute to adding new video streams. We therefore have:

$$N_{\text{streams}_{\text{CDN}}} = [\alpha + \beta \times (1 - \alpha)] \times N_{\text{streams}_{\text{DC}}} \qquad (5)$$

Equation (3) can be easily derived from (4) and (5).

The two factors α and β are important parameters of the CDN's genetic code. The problem then becomes how to derive α and β in terms of those factors in the video CDN that relate to the topology and the performance of the caching algorithms.

4 Energy Efficiency of Pervasive Wireless CDNs

Pervasive Wireless CDN concept is based on premise that entire network act as a single dispersive data centre. In today's computational paradigm

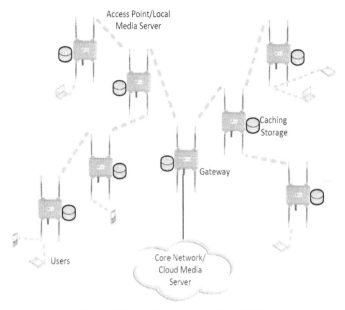

Figure 3 Pervasive mesh wireless CDN.

the microprocessor is in the centre of the computing universe and constantly shuttle data back and forth among faster and slower memories. The systems keep frequently used data close to the processor and then move it to slower and more permanent storage when it is no longer needed for the ongoing calculations [5]. Information is moved, at heavy energy cost, first to be used in computation and then stored. A parallel can be drawn with modern wireless networks, especially mesh networks, in which data is moved back and forth between the access points and application servers. The new vision, depicted in Figure 3, would be to add significant storage resources to each of the mesh AP in order to cut down on data transportation, relieve pressure on the backhaul bandwidth resources and reduce energy use.

4.1 Analytical Approach

In order to analyze energy efficiency of a pervasive wireless CDN, we simply model it as a distributed video CDN system. We assume that the pervasive mesh wireless network consists of I subnets, each subnet connected further into the network through one of I mesh gateways (i.e. $\beta = I$). We also assume a uniform user base and request pattern on each mesh-subnet. In a pervasive wireless video CDN, the intelligent content distribution algorithm pushes the most popular video content from the central media server onto the storage resources within a mesh subnet. However, this distribution of content is generally imperfect and based on probabilities. As a result, the given wireless mesh subnet will only be able to service λ of the total requests. This is known as local cache hit ratio. The hit ratio depends on the content caching algorithm, the local storage size, the service usage pattern and many other contextual parameters. Assuming the same average hit ratio is achieved at each mesh subnet within a given pervasive wireless CDN, only λ percent of concurrent requests are served from local media servers. Now, drawing a parallel with CDN analysis from the previous section, we can write the following relation:

$$N_{\text{streams}_{\text{WCDN}}} = \beta \times \lambda \times N_{\text{streams}_{\text{DC}}} \tag{6}$$

Based on equation (3), we can derive α in terms of the cache hit ratio λ:

$$\alpha = (1 - \lambda) \times \left[\frac{\beta}{\beta - 1} \right] \tag{7}$$

For the ideal case in which all the requests can be served locally, $\lambda = 1$, i.e. a 100% cache hit ratio, we have $\alpha = 0$ meaning all extra resources go to increasing the stream count by the factor of β. This is in line with the definition of α in (3). Conversely, for the worst case of $\alpha = 1$, where none of the extra resources are used to increase stream count, we have $\lambda = 1/\beta$. In that case each mesh subnet only picks up a proportional fraction of the total load. Using equations (4) and (6) we arrive at:

$$\text{efficiency}_{\text{WCDN}} = \frac{N_{\text{streams}_{\text{WCDN}}}}{E_{\text{total}_{\text{WCDN}}}} = \frac{\beta \times \lambda \times N_{\text{streams}_{\text{DC}}}}{\beta \times E_{\text{total}_{\text{DC}}}} = \lambda \times \text{efficiency}_{\text{DC}} \tag{8}$$

We can see from (8) that the efficiency of a pervasive wireless CDN, relative to a centralized network with the same amount of processing and storage resources, simply equals to the cache hit ratio of the wireless CDN local media servers. It is evident that main source of inefficiency in a pervasive wireless CDN comes from the imperfect content distribution mechanisms deployed to move, store and synchronize content across the storage/cache resources.

It can also be shown that in case of a hierarchical video CDN architecture, in which central server holds the entire content library and picks up cache misses from the pervasive wireless CDN, overall energy efficiency is still directly proportional to the hit ratio. In summary, the higher hit ratio leads to more energy efficient wireless CDN solutions.

For the reason explained above it is worthwhile to discuss possible energy efficiency improvements by means of content caching coordination across a number of subnets within a given wireless CDN.

In a pervasive wireless CDN system, several adjacent subnets can form a virtual cluster, which then cooperate in terms of coordinated caching and media synchronization in order to best accommodate usage patterns of local users.

Any improvement over the local hit ratio, due to improved media caching and synchronization strategy, will result in energy saving. In the pervasive wireless CDN system, the cache from multiple APs within a single subnet can be pooled together to form a larger, virtual storage space. Piece of video content needs to be cached only once in the virtual storage pool, by the virtualization of local media servers we can consequently host a larger video library. As presented in [8], the popularity of the cached content follows the "cut-off" Zipf-like discrete probability density distribution:

$$p_N(i) = \frac{\Omega}{i^\vartheta}, \quad \Omega = \left(\sum_{i=1}^{N} \frac{1}{i^\vartheta} \right)^{-1} \tag{9}$$

In (9), the adjusting parameter ϑ can be within $0 < \vartheta \leq 1$ range, and i is the rank order of a content title from a library of the size N. For this class of probability density functions, the hit-ratio grows in a log-like fashion as function of the cache size. A larger ϑ means more requests are concentrated on fewer hot video files. The relationship can be expressed as:

$$\lambda(S) = C \times \ln(S) \quad \text{for} \quad \vartheta = 1; \quad \lambda(S) = C \times S^{1-\vartheta} \quad \text{for} \quad 0 < \vartheta < 1 \tag{10}$$

In (10) S is the cache size and C is proportionality constant. Let us assume that there are I wireless mesh subnets (each subnet is controlled by unique Mesh GW) in a pervasive wireless CDN. Each subnet has J local media servers (i.e. APs), and the storage size of each local media server is S_{AP}. The virtual storage of a subnet is then aggregate storage across J local media servers, i.e. $S_{\text{SN}} = J \times S_{\text{AP}}$. The hit ratio for a digital library within a given subnet is:

$$\lambda_{\text{SN}} = C \times \ln(J \times S_{\text{AP}}) = \lambda + C \times \ln(J) \quad \text{for} \quad \vartheta = 1 \tag{11}$$

Or:

$$\lambda_{\text{SN}} = C \times (J \times S_{\text{AP}})^{1-\vartheta} \quad \text{for} \quad 0 < \vartheta < 1 \tag{12}$$

It is obvious that the hit ratio is to benefit from larger storage sizes on each of wireless AP and larger subnets. The concept of larger subnets can be expanded so it does not necessarily insist on the number of AP within a subnet but rather include partial content synchronization between adjacent subnets. Nevertheless, in both cases the higher hit ratio benefits energy efficiency while additional storage resources are to increase total energy consumption. Careful consideration has to be given to these two trends in order to maximize wireless CDN efficiency for the given size of content library and probability density function of content popularity.

Pervasive wireless CDN system is poised to benefit from intelligent content dispersion – i.e. partial distribution of the overall content library that turns constituting APs into localized media servers. This benefits overall energy consumption in several ways:

- APs are network elements that need to stay on regardless of their CDN assignment. Therefore, PUE and SPUE (2) parameters of APs do not significantly influence the overall system power consumption.
- Backhaul links in WMNs represent the biggest limitation in light of streaming capacity (especially those backhaul links that are closer to mesh GWs). Number of requesting users can be greater than WMN's streaming capacity (number of concurrent streams). Strategically distributing a small portion of the video content library across APs enable a certain number of requesting users to be serviced by APs to which they are directly connected. These streams will not burden the backhaul links. By intelligent load balancing over WMN backhaul links, local placement of content on APs will significantly improve streaming capacity of a pervasive wireless CDN. This will result in increased number of concurrent video streams compared to the number of streams achieved by a centralized streaming approach (parameter α decreases) and consequently bringing energy efficiency of CDN closer to that of a data center.
- Selective preloading of content on APs places it closer to the end users, consequently reducing the transport delay and access time, which in turn improves end user perceived QoS/QoE.

In the next section a replica placement algorithm is described. This algorithm makes optimal placement of required number of copies of video file, addressing transportation delay and system power consumption minimization.

4.2 Simulation Approach

A simulation model of video streaming CDN over pervasive wireless mesh network was developed to analyze merits of content caching at access points. Impact of this content caching approach on delivery tree length (which is directly proportional to transfer delay) and system power efficiency is analyzed. To tackle this problem we have modelled a CDN over pervasive wireless mesh network as a network flow problem and used a mixed integer linear programming (MILP) approach. Exact MILP problem solving is invoked within the Monte-Carlo simulation runs, in order to examine the overall cost and performance of the CDN for different replica placement cases, and number of randomly placed users/requestors, etc. Underlying network is modelled as a network flow graph with mesh type backbone graph (connection among WMN access points), with predetermined edge k-connectivity, and star topology of APs and users connected to APs. These network flow graphs, which are used for the experiments, represent discrete statistical snapshots of the network topology and user request distribution. Using Wolfram Mathematica™ and Math Works Matlab™ for generating the network graph and solving the MILP problem, we have conducted a number of distinct experiments on a CDN of varying size, whose requesting user nodes were randomly distributed across the network. Pareto-optimal (in the sense of multi-objective optimization problem at hand) replica placement strategy is calculated on basis of two key performance objectives. The first one concerns with minimization of average delivery tree length (ADTL), which is directly proportional to user perceived QoS (delay). This value is obtained by summing up the utilized router hops on the path, connecting the end user to replica server, and dividing that sum with the total number of users served. If the only goal of optimal file caching is minimization of ADTL, then parameter α from (3) will increase and come closer to 1 (it will not be equal to 1 because streaming capacity of a WMN will increase with caching on APs too). Therefore, newly deployed resources (parameter β) are meant for QoS improvement and, because of WMN technology characteristics, these new resources improve streaming capacity as well and consequently energy efficiency (see (8)). The second optimization objective is minimization of total power consumption of system. This optimization objective directly tends to improve energy efficiency of a pervasive wireless CDN system.

An MILP model of a pervasive wireless CDN system is derived from multi-commodity flow problem with multiple sources of video files (access points and source servers) and multiple sinks (requesting users). In order to

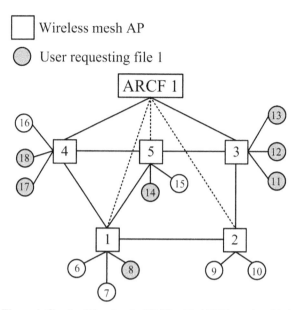

Figure 4 Graph of the simple WMN with ARCFn node added.

tackle the problem at hand we have introduced super source nodes in network flow graphs for every video file in the system (video file ⟺ commodity). Therefore, for every file, which is to be placed in the caching storage of the access points, we introduce a superficial (super source) node named All Replica Containing File n (ARCFn) and connect it to all other network nodes (parameter J from (11)) considered to be legitimate targets for placement of replica of file n.

In our experiments we have considered all WMN access points to be candidates for replica placement and the whole WMN is one subnet (all APs are connected to all GWs-directly or indirectly). Regarding these facts, ARCFn node for every file will be connected to every WMN access point in the network graph. Connecting edges are directed from ARCFn node to all candidate nodes and have weight equal to zero in order not to change the ADTL value. When needed number of copies of video file and user request distribution are derived, ARCFn node will be used as super source node, which will transform the multi-source/multi-sink multi-commodity flow problem of the original network flow graph to the single-source/multi-sink multi-commodity flow problem. Figure 4 depicts an ARCFn node concept for simple pervasive WMN network. All access points are considered to be candidates for replica placement. Therefore, there are edges from ARCF1 to all nodes representing access points. If two copies of video file 1 are to be placed in caches of WMN access points, then solid lines, representing edges from ARCF1 to access points 4 and 3, mean that these access points are selected as optimal solutions for replica placement problem.

Previously published work [2] has shown that video streaming from one centralized video server is more energy efficient then streaming from several distributed video servers. On the other hand, our results clearly show that more distributed video streaming systems have shorter ADTL and provide better QoS/QoE to the end users. Therefore power efficiency and ADTL (QoS/QoE) are two opposing requirements and optimal design of a wireless CDN will be based on the trade-off between them.

Taking into consideration multi-objective optimization problem with two optimization criteria (power consumption and ADTL) and ARCFn concept, we have formulated a MILP model of a video streaming CDN over pervasive wireless mesh network (13)–(22). Variables and parameters of the MILP model are presented in Table 1.

The MILP model is defined as:

Minimize:

$$\Sigma_f \Sigma_{(i,j)} (W \times \omega_{ij} + (1 - W) \times p''_{ij}) X^f_{ij}$$

$$+ (1 - W)(\Sigma_f \Sigma_{(k,l)} p_{kl} Q^f_{kl} + \Sigma_f \Sigma_{(k,l)} p'_{kl} Y^f_{kl})$$

$$\forall((i, j) \in (E \cup K), (k, l) \in K, f \in F), \quad 0 \le W \le 1 \quad (13)$$

Subject to:

$$\Sigma_{i,(i,k)} X^f_{ik} - \Sigma_{j,(k,j)} X^f_{kj} = L^f_k \quad \forall((i, j) \in (E \cup K), f \in F) \quad (14)$$

$$\Sigma_{(i,j)} Q^f_{ij} = N^f \quad \forall((i, j) \in K, f \in F) \quad (15)$$

$$X^f_{ij} \le M^f Y^f_{ij} \quad \forall((i, j) \in K, f \in F) \quad (16)$$

$$\Sigma_{(i,j)} Y^f_{ij} \le N^f \quad \forall((i, j) \in K, f \in F) \quad (17)$$

$$Q^f_{ij} \le q_{ij} Y^f_{ij} \quad \forall((i, j) \in K, f \in F) \quad (18)$$

$$Q^f_{ij} \ge \frac{X^f_{ij}}{M^f} \quad \forall((i, j) \in K, f \in F) \quad (19)$$

Table 1 MILP model variables and parameters.

E	Set of edges of starting CDN network
ARCFn	Virtual nodes added for delivery tree calculation convenience. ARCFn stand for "All Replica Containing File n".
K	Set of edges that are incident to ARCF nodes
F	Set of files in network
N^f	Number of copies of file f that are to be placed in network. This parameter is derived by taking into account predicted local popularity of a file and user request distribution
M^f	Total load for file f which directly equals to number of requesting users and consequently the popularity of file f
ω_{ij}	Cost of network edge (number of router hops)
L_k^f	Requested load of node k for file f
X_{ij}^f	Load for file f over edge (i, j)
Y_{ij}^f	Integer (binary) variable, encoding the existence of edge from ARCF node i for file f to replica server j
p'_{ij}	Base power consumption of network node j, encoded as (second) weight of edge between server j and ARCF node i (the first weight is ω_{ij}; for all edges starting from ARCF nodes, $\omega_{ij} = 0$). This parameter includes processing power consumed by streaming engine and caching management.
p''_{ij}	Power needed for transmitting data over wireless link
p_{ij}	Power consumption per unit of storage on network node j (unit of storage is one copy of video file)
Q_{ij}^f	Number of copies of file f stored in network node j
q_{ij}	Storage capacity of network node j. This is directly connected with the parameter β from (3) and equal to parameter S_{AP} from (11)
W	Weight coefficient for aggregation function

$$X_{ij}^f \geq 0 \quad \forall((i, j) \in (E \cup K), f \in F) \tag{20}$$

$$Q_{ij}^f \geq 0 \quad \forall((i, j) \in K, f \in F) \tag{21}$$

$$Y_{ij}^f \in \{0, 1\} \quad \forall((i, j) \in K, f \in F) \tag{22}$$

The variable Y_{ij}^f in the solution shows which of the edges between ARCFn node and corresponding candidate nodes are used in multi-commodity flow problem solution. When Y_{ij}^f equals to 1 (depicted as solid line in Figure 4), the corresponding candidate node is selected for replica placement. The variable Q_{ij}^f tells how many copies of the video file are stored in one access point. The variable X_{ij}^f shows the amount of load for every file over every edge in the network graph (number of streams going over network link). These variables compose the solution of the optimal replica placement problem. All p (p_{ij}, p'_{ij}, p''_{ij}) parameters represent different power consumptions in the system and are scaled to appropriate values (the lowest parameter receives value of 1 and others are accordingly scaled down) in order to evade the prioritization of one or the other optimization criterion.

Constraint (14) is the flow conservation for every network node. Constraint (15) represents that exactly N^f copies of file f have to be placed in the system. The maximum number of the selected nodes for replica placement is less or equal to the number of copies of file f (17). Constraint (18) represents limited storage space on APs. Constraints (16) and (19) give the connection between model variables (i.e. if Q^f_{ij} for one node is 0, then nothing can be streamed from that node, and corresponding X^f_{ij} for the edge from ARCFn to that candidate node is also 0). Domains of the variables are given in (20), (21) and (22).

Model for ADTL minimization have been developed first. For derived number of copies of video file, that are to be placed in cache space of access points, model will select all candidate nodes for replica placement if their number is less than number of copies of file. If a number of nodes (access points), which are replica candidates, exceeds number of copies of video file, model selects optimal nodes for replica placement. Objective function for optimal replica placement for purpose of ADTL minimization is:

$$\text{Minimize:} \quad \Sigma_f \Sigma_{(i,j)} \omega_{ij} X^f_{ij} \quad \forall((i,j) \in (E \cup K), f \in F) \quad (23)$$

According to the experiments, objective function (23) combined with constraints (14), (16) and (17) tends to maximally distribute copies of video file over as many access points as possible. For experimental approach described in Section 4.3 and experimental WMN graph from Figure 6, ADTL, as function of number of replica candidates, is shown in Figure 5. This confirms ADTL as optimization criterion whose minimization requires maximal decentralization of caching among WMN access points. Therefore, ADTL optimization criterion will result in energy efficiency decrease on behalf of QoS increase.

When one copy of a video file is placed on every AP in the WMN, ADTL for that file will be minimal (equal to 1 as shown in Figure 5). However, if a local popularity of that particular video file is such that streaming capacity of a WMN cannot support all stream requests, caching on more APs will increase streaming capacity of a system and consequently increase energy

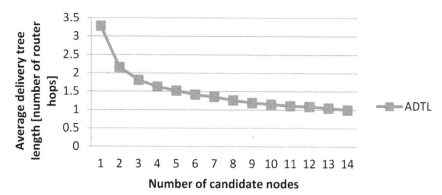

Figure 5   ADTL as function of number of candidate nodes for replica placement.

efficiency. This implies that precision of predicted local file popularity is very important for system power efficiency.

The model for minimization of system power consumption is developed in order to confirm the claims in [2], where it states that power efficiency of a video streaming CDN system goes up with streaming process centralization. The model objective function is:

$$\text{Minimize:} \quad \Sigma_f \Sigma_{(k,l)} p_{kl} Q_{kl}^f + \Sigma_f \Sigma_{(k,l)} p'_{kl} Y_{kl}^f \quad \forall ((k,l) \in K, f \in F) \quad (24)$$

Objective function (24) with constraints (15) and (17) represents MILP model for system power consumption minimization. The first sum in (24) addresses power consumption of caching storage per copy of video file. The second sum represents total base power consumption of nodes selected for replica placement. With parameter p_{kl} we can model storage devices with different power efficiency (HDD, SDD, Flash memory). Parameter p'_{kl} represents base power consumption of candidate nodes (including power needed for streaming process and caching management) and can be used for modelling data centres and devices with different power efficiency. Parameters p_{kl} and p'_{kl} directly address parameter β (3) in light of power consumption of newly deployed resources. When a number of copies of video file are derived and when we do not have storage capacity limitation on access points, power consumption minimization model will always place all copies of video file on one access point only. If all candidate nodes have the same power efficiency (base and per unit of storage power consumption), model will randomly select one candidate node. If parameters p'_{kl} and p_{kl} are different for different candidate nodes, model will select the most power efficient solution.

Power consumption of transferring video file over wireless link is the next parameter that needs to be included in the model with objective function (24). This requires that constraints (14), (16) and (19) be included into the model. By including this new system parameter, we have upgraded objective function for power consumption minimization criterion:

$$\Sigma_f \Sigma_{(i,j)} p''_{ij} X^f_{ij} + \Sigma_f \Sigma_{(k,l)} p_{kl} Q^f_{kl} + \Sigma_f \Sigma_{(k,l)} p'_{kl} Y^f_{kl} \quad \forall ((k,l) \in K, f \in F)$$
$$(25)$$

The first sum in (25) addresses power consumption for transferring video files over wireless links. This part of total system power consumption directly depends on ADTL value. With ADTL minimization, total file transferring power consumption is also minimized. Now, when the model with objective function (25) has to choose among replica candidates with the same power consumption (base and per unit of storage), it will select the one which results in minimal ADTL for requesting users. Since ADTL minimization requires caching/streaming decentralization, we come to conclusion that total system power consumption (energy efficiency) and ADTL (QoS) are not two totally opposing criteria. However, since base and storage power consumptions represent major part of the total system power consumption [9], these two optimization objectives will oppose one another and appropriate trade-off between them should be found.

Objective functions (23) and (25) represent ADTL and power consumption optimisation criterion. In order to find trade-off between these two objectives, we have combined them in one aggregated objective function. Aggregation is done with help of weight parameter W. This results in objective function (13). Parameter W (value between 0 and 1) represents importance/priority given to two different optimization criteria. Parts of the objective function (13) that are multiplied by W correspond to the ADTL optimization criterion and parts that are multiplied by $(1 - W)$ correspond to the power consumption criterion. When we want to place fixed number of copies of video file in the APs, if parameter W comes closer to value of 1, parameter α will also come closer to the value of 1. If the streaming capacity of a standard WMN is enough to serve all of the predicted user requests, then $W = 1$ results in $\alpha = 1$ (caching on APs will increase available streaming capacity of a WMN, but since user requests do not require streaming capacity increase, all new resources will be used for QoS improvement, leaving number of served users the same as for the original WMN). When streaming capacity of a standard WMN is not enough to serve all requesting users, $W = 1$ will result in $\alpha < 1$, because number of concurrent streams will increase with caching on APs. By taking into account power consumption, as one of the optimization criterion for optimal replica placement, when parameter W tends to a value of 0, parameter α will also tend to a value of 0.

The next step in MILP model evolution is adding the storage capacity constraint (18). When caching storage of APs has unlimited capacity, all copies of video file, which need to be placed into the system, can be stored on one AP. In reality, APs will have very limited storage capacity, which will make candidate nodes selection more challenging problem from power consumption objective point of view. Experiments were conducted in order to determine influence of the storage size of APs on the power consumption of the system as well as on the ADTL and establish the trade-off dependency between them.

As discussed in [9], CDN systems using caching of content at networking elements (routers, access points, etc.) achieve greater energy efficiency than those with centralized streaming approach. This claim from [9] is based on the fact that networking elements work all the time (regardless whether or not they are streaming video content), therefore their base power consumption should not be included in power consumption of the overall CDN system. Furthermore, the content cached on access points is being placed closer to the end users, which results in shorter ADTL and consequently the improvement of the QoS perceived by the users.

Spatial user request distribution and weight factors for both of the optimization criterions are the inputs into the optimization algorithm (13)–(22) which in turn produces a pareto-optimal replica placement. The model assumptions are: (a) all access points have the same power consumption per unit of storage, (b) one unit of storage is equivalent to the video file size, (c) additional power required to run local media server services is identical from AP to AP, (d) all APs poses the same storage capacity, and (e) transmission power consumption is the same for all wireless links in the system.

4.3 Experiments

Wireless mesh network used in this experiment is shown in Figure 6. It is a wireless mesh network with k-connected mesh backbone where $k = 2$, which permits multiple paths between APs. This makes network graph more realistic, since a good wireless mesh structure, in practice, requires for every access point to be able to connect to multiple neighbouring APs. The rectangles represent wireless access points and all of them are candidates for replica placement. Shaded circles depict users that are requesting the

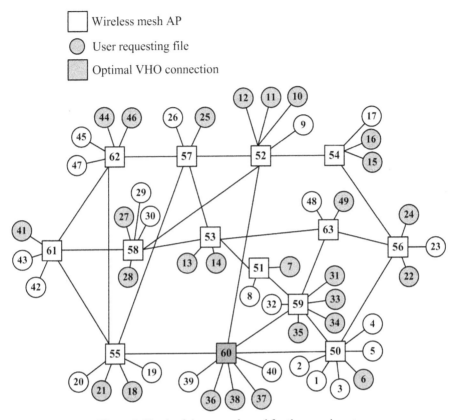

Figure 6 Graph of the network used for the experiment.

video file. The shaded rectangle represents optimal connection for video server for the case of centralized video streaming. This solution is used for benchmarking the other solutions.

As mentioned earlier, base power consumption of APs does not need to be included into the overall CDN system power consumption. On the other hand, streaming/caching servers are dedicated devices and as such all of their power consumption goes directly to the overall CDN system power consumption. Speaking in relative power units, as used in this experiment, power consumption of a streaming server (shaded rectangle in Figure 6) is around 400 which is at least 4 times more than the most power consuming scenario (only ADTL minimization is considered, see Figure 8) when streaming is done only from WMN access points.

Table 2 Content distribution among access points with changes of parameter W.

W	50	51	52	53	54	55	56	57	58	59	60	61	62	63	ADTL	Power
0	0	0	0	0	3	4	0	0	3	4	0	0	0	0	1.63	78
0.1	0	0	4	0	0	3	0	0	0	3	0	0	0	4	1.63	78
0.2	0	0	0	0	3	4	0	0	3	4	0	0	0	0	1.63	78
0.3	0	0	0	0	3	4	0	0	3	4	0	0	0	0	1.63	78
0.4	0	0	3	0	0	0	0	0	0	2	3	0	3	3	1.52	80
0.5	0	0	2	0	2	2	0	0	2	3	3	0	0	0	1.41	82
0.6	0	0	1	2	2	2	2	0	0	2	2	0	1	0	1.26	88
0.7	0	0	1	1	1	1	2	0	2	2	2	0	2	0	1.18	91
0.8	1	1	1	1	1	1	1	1	1	1	1	1	1	1		111
0.9	1	1	1	1	1	1	1	1	1	1	1	1	1	1		111
1	1	1	1	1	1	1	1	1	1	1	1	1	1	1		111

When $W = 1$, only ADTL minimization is considered and for $W = 0$ minimization of the system power consumption is the only optimization goal. In the simulation trials, for each value of access point storage capacity, we vary the W parameter over the whole range of [0, 1] with steps of 0.1 in order to gain a better understanding of the trade-off between the ATDL and power consumption. In Table 2 it is shown how copies of file are distributed among access points with parameter W changing.

The experimental task was to place 14 copies (the number of access points) of file into the access points caching storages whose capacity is 5. For lower parameter W values, power consumption is more dominant optimization criterion and therefore model tends to place number of requested copies over as minimal number of access points as possible. Replica placement, in cases when parameter W takes values from 0 to 0.3 (see Table 2), results in the same power consumption and ADTL values, although selected candidate nodes are not the same. In cases like this MILP model will randomly select one of the solutions. From $W = 0.4$ to $W = 0.7$, replica placement solution changes with every step resulting in increased value of power consumption and decrease in ADTL value. The last three values of W parameter from Table 2 result in replica placement solution where one copy of video file is placed on every access point. This results in minimal value of ADTL and maximal value of system power consumption.

Including more access points in the streaming process impose greater power inefficiency than placing more copies on the same access point. By including power consumed for content transmission into MILP model, more realistic results are obtained. For example, in the case when $W = 0$ we have streaming from four access points, although their caching capacity allows for

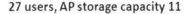

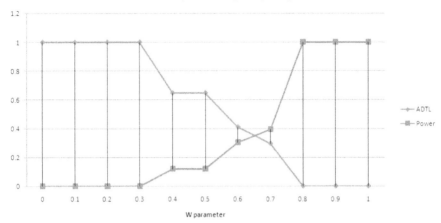

Figure 7 ADTL and power consumption are two opposed optimisation criteria.

streaming to be done from three access points. Streaming from three access points is better from a power consumption point of view if the delivery tree length (transmission power consumption) is not included into the overall system power consumption model. However, streaming from four access points results in sufficient ADTL reduction that overall system power consumption is actually minimized by including additional AP into the streaming process. This is the result of transmission power consumption being included in the experiment. The last two columns from the right in Table 2 show how ADTL decreases and power consumption increases with growing parameter W.

From the results of this experiment we can see that minimization of power consumption and ADTL are two opposed optimization criteria, see Figure 7. Opposing nature of these two performance parameters can be seen in Figure 8 which depicts how increase in AP storage capacity impacts the overall system power consumption and ADTL. When available storage resource on an AP is limited, the hit ratio (λ) is low and a significant amount of AP resources will be used for relaying video streams, which results in power consumption increase. However, since we have to place the precise number of copies of video files in the storage of APs, a lower level of AP storage capacity results in a decrease of the ADTL. With growth of storage capacity of the APs, the replica placement algorithm has greater freedom in determining how many APs to include into the streaming process and which ones, resulting in power consumption minimization.

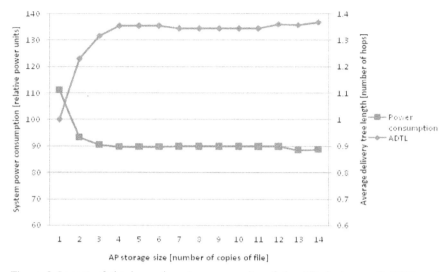

Figure 8 Impact of the increasing storage capacity of the APs in terms of ADTL and consumed power metrics.

We can see from Figure 8 that after a certain threshold, there is no benefit in adding additional storage resources, as they are not improving the hit ratio and consequently the changes in ADTL and power consumption are negligible.

5 Conclusion

In this paper we have investigated the energy efficiency of a special class of video CDN system, namely pervasive wireless CDN based on Mesh Wi-Fi implementation. Both analytical calculations and computer simulations confirmed our initial hypothesis that content placement strategy for a wireless CDN has to carefully balance energy consumption versus QoS/latency performances. We have captured the idea of intelligent coordination of content placement among wireless access points that serve as edge video servers into a number of experiments. Computer simulations are conducted based on mixed integer linear programming (MILP) model in order to demonstrate its capability to come up with pareto-optimal content placement and caching strategies as function of power consumption and QoS requirements. Our analytical approach has shown very strong dependency between the energy efficiency for this class of CDNs and associated content hit ratio. All of this points out towards a very strong need to build a context driven wireless video delivery networks in which content/caching placement strategies are dynamically changed in accordance with user's request changes, user's mobility and content popularity.

References

[1] Gerhard Fettweis and Ernesto Zimmermann. ICT Energy Consumption – Trends and Challenges. In *Proceedings of the 11th International Symposium on Wireless Personal Multimedia Communications (WPMC 2008)*.
[2] Dragan Boscovic, Michael Needham, Faramak Vakil, and Jin Yang. Low Carbon Economy Considerations in Designing and Operating Content Delivery Networks for VoD Services. *Journal of Green Engineering*, 1(1):33–53, 2010.
[3] Ning Xu, Jin Yang, Mike Needham, Dragan Boscovic, and Faramak Vakil. Toward the Green Video CDN. In *Proceedings IEEE/ACM International Conference on Green Computing*, Hangshou, Zhejiang Province, China, 18 December 2010.
[4] Terry Cudmore and Cris Nicoll. Preparing for 4G Video Services, Yankee Group, 30 July 2010.
[5] Remapping Computer Circuitry to Avert Impending Bottlenecks. http://www.nytimes.com/2011/03/01/science/01compute.hml?_r=3&ref=science.
[6] Green Grid Metrics: Describing Data Center Power Efficiency. White paper, www.greengrid.org, January 2007.
[7] B.L. Buzbee. The Efficiency of Parallel Processing. Frontiers of Supercomputing. *Los Alamos Science*, 71, 1983.
[8] L. Breslau et al. Web caching and Zipf-Like distributions: Evidence and implications. In *Proceedings of IEEE INFOCOMM 99*, pages 21–25, March 1999.
[9] V. Valancius, N. Laoutaris, L. Massoulie, C. Diot, and P. Rodriguez. Greening the Internet with Nano Data Centers. In *Proceedings of ACM CoNEXT'09*, Rome, Italy, 1–4 December 2009.

Biographies

Dragan Boscovic heads Core Research activities for Motorola Mobility Inc. As senior director Boscovic leads a talented team of researchers that identify opportunities for new products, systems and services. His team leverages internet technologies and services to create solution architectures for context driven applications such as Social TV, media sharing, and adaptive video streaming over fixed and wireless networks. Migration of service enablers toward home platforms such as home gateways, set-tops, WiFi access points and cellular CPE devices in context of the Wireless Healthcare is another area of particular interest.

Prior to this role, Boscovic served as director of Engineering and Technology for Motorola's Strategic Growth Engine, where he developed technologies that enhanced consumer's abilities to connect with multimedia and one another. He also worked within Motorola's R&D sites in Europe for 12 years. Boscovic is known for his work on Radio Ecology, which describes better use of the limited resources of the radio frequency (RF) spectrum. His vision in this domain led to a number of large collaborative research programs in Europe. He is also credited with the vision of Cognitive Networks which he published in 2005 and is being further developed by wider research community ever since.

Boscovic has amassed 22 patents, with eight more pending, and has published numerous papers on topics including wireless technologies and cognitive networks. He is often called upon to share insights on wireless topics at industry events such as the International Consumer Electronic Show, Global Semiconductor Forum, AlwaysOn, Wireless World Initiative and Wireless World Research Forum.

Boscovic received his Bachelor's and Master's degrees from the University of Belgrade in Serbia and his doctorate degree from the University of Bath in the UK.

Faramak Vakil is a Distinguished Member of Technical Staff in the Motorola Applied Research Center working on network and service management. Prior to joining Motorola in 2006, he was a Senior Scientist in the Applied Research Area of Telcordia. He received his Ph.D. degree in Electrical Engineering from Columbia University in the City of New York in 1984, and immediately joined Bellcore (now Telcordia).

Since 1998, Faramak has almost exclusively focused on the architecture, design, control and management of a mobile Internet. He has devised novel mobility, network self-organization and management, and service creation schemes for a mobile Internet. From 1993–1997, he worked on performance management of ATM networks; where he led the design and implementation of an ATM monitoring system, devised a self-assembling network simulator, and conducted experimental studies on the performance of TCP/IP over ATM in hybrid terrestrial-satellite networks. From 1987–1993, he exclusively worked on the specifications of ATM protocols where he developed the error, flow and congestion control; as well as circuit emulation and service clock recovery mechanisms for ATM. In his first assignment, 1984–1986, he devised a performance monitoring system for the Bellcore MAN trials in Boston and New York. Faramak is a member of ACM and IEEE. He has published numerous papers and standard contributions, and has several patents.

Staniša Dautović is an assistant professor and senior researcher within the Department of Power, Electronics and Communications Engineering, Faculty of Technical Sciences, University of Novi Sad, Serbia. He received the Ph.D. degree in Electrical Engineering from University of Novi Sad, Serbia in 2009. His research interest is oriented towards combinatorial optimization and applied algorithms in engineering, theory of algorithms and complexity, formal verification of digital and analog circuits, algorithms for VLSI design automation, parallel and distributed algorithms for multiprocessor and multicore systems. He is currently a member of the Embedded Systems & Algorithms research group. Dautovic is a member of IEEE, and author or co-author of nine scientific papers.

Milenko Tošić is a research engineer at La Citadelle Inzenjering Novi Sad. He received his Master of Science degree in Electrical Engineering from University of Novi Sad, Serbia 2009. He is currently pursuing a Ph.D. degree at Department of Power, Electronics and Communications Engineering, Faculty of Technical Sciences, University of Novi Sad, Serbia. His research interest is oriented towards knowledge based computer network management, context aware algorithms and protocols for radio communication, wireless mesh network specific protocols and algorithms, multimedia content conditioning and adaptation and opportunistic networking.

Energy Efficiency in Cognitive Radio Network

P.S.M. Tripathi and Ramjee Prasad

Centre for Teleinfrastructure (CTiF), Aalborg University, Aalborg, Denmark;
e-mail: in_psmt@es.aau.dk

Received 12 September 2011; Accepted: 25 September 2011

Abstract

In recent years, green communications has received a lot of attention in academic society. Cognitive radio techniques have been introduced to improve the spectrum utilization in already allocated spectrum band to licensed user as well as it promotes green communications. Under spectrum sharing model, secondary users can share spectrum with primary users under condition that total interference caused by SUs should not be exceeded from a predefined level. Energy efficiency is one of the important metric in cognitive radio network as it has to work under strict transmit power constraint. In this paper we explore how better energy efficiency can be achieved in spectrum sharing environment. Our analysis shows that energy efficiency in cognitive radio network is better when number of secondary users is more than available channels.

Keywords: cognitive radio, quality of service, power control, spectrum sharing, energy efficiency.

1 Introduction

Other than economy aspects, spectrum scarcity and green communications are two serious challenges that nowadays wireless industry is facing. It is well-known fact that wireless based services can survive only when desired spectrum is available and consume less power. Cognitive radio [1, 2] is considered a promising technology which can deal both problems simultaneously.

In the recent years, with the emergence of new wireless services, demand for the spectrum has been increased manyfold. Radio spectrum is a natural scarce resource and most of the useful portion has already been allotted to various services and regulators are facing difficulties to accommodate new wireless services in the desired frequency band. Studies on spectrum utilization have shown the different picture. Studies shows that spectrum is underutilized in most of the frequency bands at given time and location meaning that, part of the frequency band could be free and available at a particular time and location, although it has been allocated to some primary services [3]. The Federal Communication Commission (FCC) [4] estimates that the variation of use of licensed spectrum ranges from 15 to 85%, while Defence Advance Research Projects Agency (DARPA) [3] claims that only 2% of the spectrum is in use in the US at any given moment, even if all bands are allocated.

Green communication is basically intended to reduce CO_2 emissions to protect the environment. Wireless industry is growing very fast, new technologies are coming very fast and surpassing old technology with higher data transfer rate and converging more and more services at one platform. In this process total energy consumption by the communication devices are also increasing significantly 16–20% per annum, almost doubles every five years. According to a climate report on Green Communications [5]

> Currently 3% of the worldwide energy is consumed by the ICT (Information & Communications Technology) infrastructure that causes about 2% of the worldwide CO_2 emissions, which is comparable to the worldwide CO_2 emissions by airplanes or one quarter of the worldwide CO_2 emissions by cars.

Therefore, lowering energy consumption of future wireless radio systems are demanding greater attention and requires new technologies and solutions and is becoming an important factor in specification of future standards [6]. Cognitive radio technology initially designed to cope with spectrum scarcity, but due to its inherent properties like strict energy constraint and opportunistic spectrum sharing with primary users without causing harmful interference makes it ideal for green communications as well. Cognitive Radio is characterized of an adaptive, multidimensionally aware, autonomous radio system empowered by advanced intelligent functionality, which interacts with its operating environment and learns from its experiences to reason, plan, and decide future actions to meet various needs [7]. This approach leads to a significant increase in spectrum efficiency, networking efficiency as well as energy efficiency. Benefits of cognitive radio with respect to green communications are presented in [7, 8].

In cognitive radio network, unlicensed secondary users (SUs) are allowed to share the same spectrum along with the licensed primary user (PU) as long as interference generated by SUs is below the acceptable noise floor for the PU of the spectrum as decided by the regulator. Restriction on transmitted power by SU can be compensated allowing them to gain access wide bandwidth [9]. This approach is known as spectrum sharing or underlay approach. Power control in SUs network play one of the most important factors in cognitive radio network. There are two main categories of power control in CR networks: (a) centralized power control [10, 11], where a central manager controls the transmission power of all users within its coverage area; (b) distributed power control [11, 12] where each user controls its transmission power by itself using only local information. However, since the interference temperature at the PU receiver cannot be identified by the local information, it is difficult that the QoS requirement for the PU is guaranteed in the distributed power control. In [12], the authors proposed a fully autonomous distributed power control scheme without an additional process for CR networks where the constraint for the sum of the interference induced by all SUs in the network is replaced by a new constraint which limits the individual transmission power by making the strong assumption that the total interference constraint at the PU caused by all SUs is divided equally between SUs. As cognitive radio is in nascent stage, centralised control is easier to maintain. It has the advantage of easing the regulator's control of spectrum usage, and allowing them to direct how the spectrum is used [13].

In communication system, performance can be measured in different ways. At the lowest level, bit error rate (BER) is basic criteria to measure the performance of the link. Another criteria goodput or application level throughput measures the amount of usable bits that received by the link [14]. These metrics provide an extremely low level and detailed view of the performance of a communications system. According to the Shannon equation [15] Goodput is related to bandwidth and transmitted power. In [16], a variable power and bandwidth efficient modulation strategy has been discussed. It has been shown that channel capacity can be enhanced by maximising bandwidth efficiency, but this constantly increases the complexity of the system which increases the overhead of the network. Another option is that if bandwidth is kept constant, goodput is dependent on transmitted power. High goodput means high transmit power though increment is not linear. If we wish to minimize transmitted power, we have to compromise on goodput for a given bandwidth. A trade-off is needs to be done depending on the situation. In this paper, a trade-off between transmit power and goodput in a centralised cognitive radio network is investigated from the aspect of energy efficiency. This is an extension of our previous work [17]. We also investigate what would be the impact on energy efficiency if the number of available channels is limited as compared to SUs.

The rest of this paper is organised as follows: Section 2 describes the system model, performance metrics and our main assumptions. In Section 3, simulation environment and results are analyzed and finally, conclusions are discussed in Section 4.

2 System Model and Performance Metrics

We consider a spectrum-sharing model in which secondary users are allowed to use the same spectrum licensed to a primary user simultaneously as long as interference level at primary user receiver is within predefined level. Assume that N pairs of SUs devices (a transmitter and its corresponding receiver) distributed in an area away from PU receiver and far away from PU transmitter such that interference due to PU transmitter at SUs receiver is negligible. The links between SUs and between SUs & PU receiver are flat Rayleigh fading channels. In Rayleigh fading channels, the channel power gains are exponentially distributed and have a mean values which depends on distance from PU and SU transmitters and also from distance between SUs transmitters and receivers. We also consider that channel state information between receiver & transmitter of the secondary users and primary receiver & secondary transmitters are perfectly known to SUs through a central band manager, which mediates between primary and secondary users. We will use the following notations in the paper: $g_{i,i}$ is the channel gain between the ith SU transmitter and its corresponding receiver, $g_{i,j}$ is the channel gain between the ith SU transmitter and the jth SU receiver and $g_{PU,i}$ is the channel gain between the ith SU transmitter and PU receiver. P_i is peak transmit power from the ith SU and I_{max} is the maximum predefined tolerable interference level at the PU receiver.

A reliable implementation of cognitive radio network depends not only upon the maximum tolerable interference level at primary receiver but also on transmitted power of secondary user which determined by its target SNR.

These two constraints are considered as quality of service (QoS) requirement in cognitive radio network.

2.1 Threshold Interference Level at Primary Receiver

PU will always maintain its threshold SNR irrespective of how many SUs enter into the network and share the same spectrum. The total interference caused by SUs at PU receiver should always be less than to a predefined level $I_{\max}$. The QoS requirement for the primary receiver can be expressed as:

$$\sum_{i=0}^{N} g_{\text{PU},i} P_i \leq I_{\max} \tag{1}$$

2.2 Target SNR of SUs

A secondary user's received signal to noise ratio (SNR) at its receivers at which it received data from its corresponding transmitter, constitutes the secondary user QoS. SNR of the ith SU receiver is given as follows:

$$\gamma_i = \frac{g_{i,i}(t) P_i(t)}{\sum_{j=1, j \neq i}^{N} g_{i,j} P_j(t) + N_0 B} \tag{2}$$

where N_0 is the power spectral density of the AWGN noise and B represents the received signal bandwidth. P_i is the power level of the ith SU. $g_{i,i}$ is the channel gain between the ith SU transmitter & receiver and $g_{i,j}$ is the channel gain between the jth SU transmitter and the ith SU receiver. Assuming that all SUs are working on the same threshold SNR (γ_{th}), reliable communication would occur only when

$$\gamma_i \geq \gamma_{\text{th}} \tag{3}$$

Considering the QoS requirement as given in Eq. (2) for SUs, Eq. (2) can be expressed as

$$P_i \geq \gamma_{\text{th}} \left(\sum_{j=1, j \neq i}^{N} \frac{g_{i,j} P_j}{g_{i,i}} + \frac{N_0 B}{g_{i,i}} \right) \tag{4}$$

Let vector $\mathbf{P} = (P_1, P_1, P_1, \ldots, P_N)^T$ denote the transmit powers of the users. Eq. (5) can be rewritten with equality in matrix form as follows:

$$(\mathbf{I} - \mathbf{F})\mathbf{P} = \mathbf{U} \tag{5}$$

where $\mathbf{I}$ is $N \times N$ identity matrix, $\mathbf{F}$ is $N \times N$ and $\mathbf{U}$ is $N \times 1$ matrix, being specified as

$$\mathbf{F(i, j)} = \begin{cases} \gamma_{\text{th}} \frac{g_{i,j}}{g_{i,i}}, & i \neq j \\ 0, & i = j \end{cases} \tag{6}$$

$$\mathbf{U} = \gamma_{\text{th}} \frac{N_0 B}{G_{i,i}} \tag{7}$$

If the maximum eigenvalue of matrix $\mathbf{F}$ is less than 1, there exist a non-negative $\mathbf{P}$, which satisfies Eq. (5). The required threshold SNR is achievable with $\mathbf{P^*} = (\mathbf{I} - \mathbf{F})^{-1}\mathbf{U}$ being the Pareto optimal solution and the system is feasible [12]. However, the SUs cannot increase their transmission power indefinitely; there must be an upper limit for SUs transmitted power as

$$0 \leq P_i \leq P_{\text{peak}} \quad \text{for all SUs} \tag{8}$$

Secondary users can make communication when their transmit power requirements satisfy Eq. (8). If the total interference level at primary user receiver would be above the predefined level, some of the secondary users would go off. In any case enormously high power cannot be transmitted by secondary users in cognitive radio network. This shows that a cognitive radio network is more energy efficient as compared to a primary licensed network.

2.3 Performance Metrics

The choice of the proper performance metric to measure the efficiency of the power management strategy in terms of average energy consumption requires some preliminary considerations. A better definition of the energy efficiency is the one used in [8, 18]. However, this definition is not very useful when the transmission is not continuous in time. A better definition of energy efficiency for system where transmission is not continuous can be described average goodput over per unit average transmitted power. This can be given by

$$\eta = \frac{g_d}{P_{\text{total}}} \tag{9}$$

where P_{total} is the average total power transmitted by SUs and g_d is the average goodput produced by SUs. Goodput is the number of bits successfully transmitted in one second by SUs [14] and it can be written as follows:

$$\text{Goodput}(g_d) = \frac{r(t_1 + t_2 + \cdots + t_n)}{T}(1 - P_e)r \tag{10}$$

where r is the data rate in bit/s; T is the packet duration; P_e is the Packet Error Rate (PER) and t_i is the time interval in which the ith SU is transmitting during the time interval T.

Energy efficiency also depends upon the modulation scheme. A high level modulation scheme means more power whereas a low rate modulation scheme means low transmit power and better efficiency [16].

3 Results and Discussion

In this section, we assume that two fixed secondary users are allowed to use the same spectrum licensed to a primary user under spectrum-sharing model. For simulation, we assume a packet length of 200 bits and a data rate of 100 Kbps BPSK transmission in 100 KHz bandwidth. At given transmit power, first preference will be given to both users transmit simultaneously. If not possible preference will be given user which transmits less power. If these two cases are not possible within given transmit power and interference constraint, both the SUs will go off. We consider that both SUs are 400m apart and their proximity from primary receiver is 200 m. The distance between secondary transmitter and receiver is 100 m.

The relationship between packet error rate (PER), probability error (p_e), target SNR depends upon the modulation/coding scheme and the data rate. Assuming a binary phaseshift keying (BPSK) modulation scheme and no coding with N_p is the number of packets per second, the relationship among goodput and PER can be expressed as

$$p_e = \frac{1}{2}\text{erfc}\left\{\sqrt{(\text{SNR}_{\text{threshold}})}\right\} \tag{11}$$

$$\text{PER} = 1 - (1 - p_e)^{N_p} \tag{12}$$

Under spectrum sharing model in cognitive radio network, two quality of services (QoS) requirement i.e., threshold SNR in SUs network and maximum interference at PU receiver need to be satisfied simultaneously. Under normal circumstances, average goodput in SUs channel increases with increasing peak transmit power, reaches to maximum and no further increment is visible while increasing peak transmit power. The goodput variation with peak power at different threshold SNR value is shown in Figure 1.

At low peak power, goodput is low because threshold SNR criteria is difficult to meet whereas at high peak power, goodput is almost constant due to predefined maximum interference level at PU receiver. It restricts the fur-

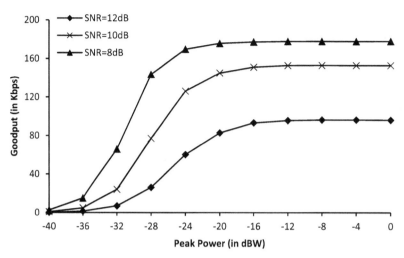

Figure 1   Goodput versus peak power at $I_{max} = -110$ dBW.

ther increase in average goodput and at this stage secondary network is under saturation condition. Therefore, maximum interference level at PU receiver is dominant constraint at high peak power. If we look at energy efficiency curve, efficiency decreases with increasing peak transmit power and after at certain level, it becomes almost constant irrespective of peak transmit power. At high peak power, interference level criteria put a cap over SUs participation due to which efficiency becomes almost constant. The energy efficiency variation with peak power at different threshold SNR value is shown in Figure 2. It is also shown that there is no significant variation in energy efficiency at different threshold SNR value though a clear variation in goodput can be seen.

Energy efficiency is the ratio of average goodput and peak power and this ratio is almost constant at different SNR as average goodput and sum of average peak power both increase simultaneously while lowering SNR. It is also shown that there is no significant variation in energy efficiency at different threshold SNR value though a clear variation in goodput. Energy efficiency is the ratio of average goodput and peak power and this ratio is almost constant at different SNR as average goodput and sum of peak power in one simulation cycle, both increases simultaneously while lowering SNR.

Average goodput and energy efficiency at two peak transmits power -32 and -24 dBW at 10 dB SNR under strict interference level at PU receiver (I_{max}) are shown in Figure 3. At low peak power, efficiency is high, but

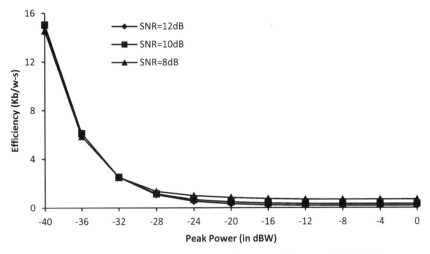

Figure 2 Energy efficiency versus peak power at $I_{max} = -110$ dBW.

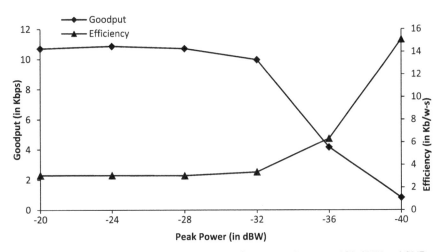

Figure 3 Energy efficiency and goodput versus peak power at $I_{max} = -123$ dBW and SNR = 10 dB.

goodput is low whereas at high peak power goodput is high and efficiency is low, but both are almost constant. Selection of peak power is depending upon what we need to achieve. At very high peak power, there is no significant increment or decrement in goodput as well as in energy efficiency. Therefore, high peak power is not advisable in cognitive radio network. It also restricts

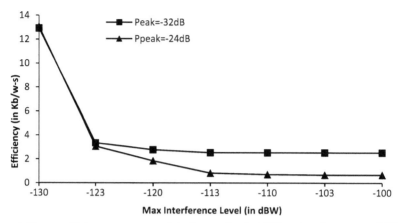

Figure 4 Energy efficiency versus max interference level at different peak power and SNR is 10 dB.

the participation of number of SUs. On the other hand choosing low peak power is also not advisable though energy efficiency is very high, but goodput is very low. Low peak power is suitable when we have to transfer small amount of data. Neither too high nor too low peak power is an ideal situation in cognitive radio network because goodput and energy efficiency both are moderate.

The interference level at primary user receiver is the most important criteria in cognitive radio network. Energy efficiency at different interference levels at two different peak transmit powers is shown in Figure 4. At a very high interference level, energy efficiency is very high due to low peak power. As we decrease the value of the interference level, energy efficiency decreases and attains almost a constant value. This shows the saturation state at a given peak transmit power. The situation will change when we change the peak transmit power.

Now we increase the number of SUs at a peak power of -32 dBW and 10 dB SNR under the same conditions. The variation in energy efficiency with respect to the number of SUs at different interference levels is shown in Figure 5. It shows that the energy efficiency increases with an increasing number of SUs at a given interference level. The energy efficiency is higher under strict interference conditions due to a low average peak power. As we increase the number of SUs, channel occupancy increases resulting in higher goodput and more power consumption, but the increment in goodput is more than the power consumption due to the interference limit which gives a high

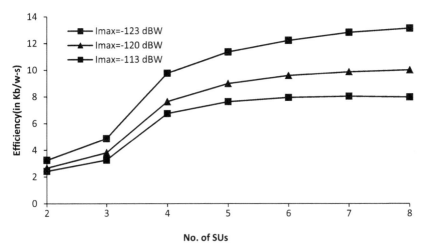

Figure 5 Energy efficiency versus the number of SUs at different interference levels. Peak power is −32 dBW and SNR is 10 dB.

energy efficiency. A high interference limit means less power consumption and a high energy efficiency.

In the next scenario, we consider that only two channels are available for SUs communications and at a time only two SUs having the lowest possible peak power for communication. Variation in energy efficiency with respect to the number of SUs under such conditions is shown in Figure 6 where the energy efficiency with respect to the number of SUs under these two conditions at 123 dBW interference level has been shown. Under strict interference conditions, the energy efficiency is almost equal when the number of SUs is less than 5 but when we increase the number of SUs beyond 5, energy efficiency increases as compared to the situation when there is no cap on the number of channels.

This increment in energy efficiency is more visible when interference condition is more relaxed. This can be seen in Figure 7, where the energy efficiency with respect to the number of SUs under similar conditions at −110 dBW interference level has been shown. The difference in energy efficiency is clearly visible in two different conditions. Restricting two SUs at a time, the average goodput is lower than in a normal situation and the average power consumption is lower which gives better energy efficiency. It shows that channel utilisation in terms of energy efficiency is high when the number of SUs is higher than the number of available channels. This also gives better spectrum utilisation.

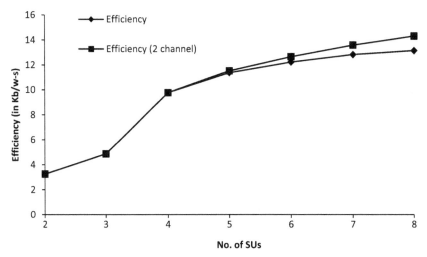

Figure 6 Comparison of the energy efficiency in normal conditions and two channel conditions at $I_{\max} = -123$ dBW. Peak power is -32 dBW and SNR is 10 dB.

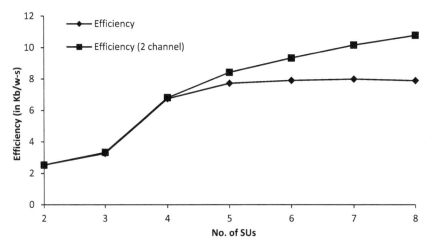

Figure 7 Comparison of the energy efficiency in normal conditions and two channel conditions at $I_{\max} = -110$ dBW. Peak power is -32 dBW and SNR is 10 dB.

4 Conclusions

We have presented the energy efficiency in cognitive radio networks for multiple secondary users under a centralised power allocation scheme. The simulation result shows that the average energy efficiency is better at low peak transmit power, but goodput is very low. Therefore, a slightly higher peak power is better because goodput and energy efficiency both are moderate and data transfer can be made effectively. This also provides more SUs participation simultaneously, allowing a lower use of batteries in a device and a better spectrum utilisation. Energy efficiency and spectrum utilisation can further be enhanced when the number of SUs is more than the available channels. There is one disadvantage, which is that data transmission by SUs may not be continuous due to the limited number of available channels as compared to the number of SUs trying to communicate. Therefore, delay is inevitable in SUs transmission under such conditions. This scenario is suitable for application such as WLAN, where continuous data transfer is not required whereas applications like voice communication may not be suitable for such a scenario. The energy efficiency can be further increased by a tradeoff between peak power, SNR and bandwidth. A field approach to such scenario would be more interesting and could be the subject of further research work.

References

[1] J. Mitola, III and G. Q. Maguire, Jr. Cognitive Radio: Making Software Radios More Personal. *IEEE, Personal Communications*, 6:13–18, 1999.

[2] S. Haykin. Cognitive Radio: Brain-Empowered Wireless Communications. *IEEE Journal on Selected Areas in Communications*, 23:201–220, 2005.

[3] M. Gandetto, A. F. Cattoni, and C. S. Regazzoni. A Distributed Approach to Mode Identification and Spectrum Monitoring for Cognitive Radios. Available: http://www.sdrforum.org/pages/sdr05/4.3%20Spectrum%20Mgmt%20and%20 Cognitive%20Radio%201/4.3-02%20Gandetto%20et%20al.pdf.

[4] FCC, ET Docket No 03-222 Notice of Proposed Rulemaking and Order. December 2003.

[5] SMART2020: Enabling the Low Carbon Economy in the Information Age. In *The Climate Group SMART 2020 Report*, June 2008.

[6] Workshop on W-GREEN. Available: http://www.wireless-world-research.org/fileadmin/ sites/default/files/meetings/Available:Related%20Events/Workshop_on_W-Green.pdf.

[7] Y.-S. Chen. Wireless Communication via Cognitive Dimension. Available: www.csie.ntpu.edu.tw/~yschenAvailable:/course/99-2/WMN/WMN_ch7.pdf.

[8] Gürkan Gür and Fatih Alagöz. Green wireless communications via cognitive dimension: an overview, *IEEE Network*, 25:50–56, 2011.

[9] S. Srinivasa and S. A. Jafar. The Throughput Potential of Cognitive Radio: A Theoretical Perspective. In *Proceedings of Fortieth Asilomar Conference on Signals, Systems and Computers (ACSSC'06)*, pages 221–225, 2006.

[10] H. S. T. Le and L. Qilian. An Efficient Power Control Scheme for Cognitive Radios. In *Proceedings of Wireless Communications and Networking Conference (WCNC2007)*, pages 2559–2563, IEEE, 2007.

[11] W. Wei, P. Tao, and W. Wenbo. Optimal Power Control Under Interference Temperature Constraints in Cognitive Radio Network. In *Proceedings of Wireless Communications and Networking Conference (WCNC2007)*, pages 116–120, IEEE, 2007.

[12] I. Sooyeol, H. Jeon, and L. Hyuckjae. Autonomous Distributed Power Control for Cognitive Radio Networks. In *Proceedings of IEEE 68th Vehicular Technology Conference (VTC2008)*, pages 1–5, 2008.

[13] L. Berlemann, S. Mangold, and A. Jarosch. Operator Assisted Cognitive Radio for Dynamic Spectrum Access and Spectrum Sharing. In *Proceedings of Wireless World Research Forum 17 (WWRF17)*, Heidelberg, Germany, November 2006.

[14] A. Amanna, T. Tsou, X. Chen, D. Datla, T. R. Newman, J. H. Reed, and T. Bose. Green Communications: A New Paradigm for Creating Cost Effective Wireless Systems. Available: http://filebox.vt.edu/users/aamanna/web%20page/Green%20Communications-draft%20journal%20paper.pdf.

[15] C. E. Shannon. Communication in the Presence of Noise. *Proceedings of the IEEE*, 72:1192–1201, 1984.

[16] D. Grace, C. Jingxin, J. Tao, and P. D. Mitchell. Using Cognitive Radio to Deliver "Green" Communications. In *Proceedings of 4th International Conference on Cognitive Radio Oriented Wireless Networks and Communications (CROWNCOM'09)*, pages 1–6, 2009.

[17] P. S. M. Tripathi, E. Cianca, M. D. Sanctis, M. Ruggieri, and R. Prasad. Truncated Power Control over Cognitive Radio Networks: Trade-off Capacity/Energy Efficiency. Paper presented at the 13th International Symposium on Wireless Personal Multimedia Communication (WPMC), Brazil, 2010.

[18] C. U. Saraydar, N. B. Mandayam, and D. J. Goodman. Efficient Power Control via Pricing in Wireless Data Networks. *IEEE Transactions on Communications*, 50:291–303, 2002.

Biographies

P.S.M. Tripathi is an Indian Engineering Services officer of the 1998 batch. He has over 10 years of technical experience in the field of Radio Communications/Radio Spectrum Management. He is Engineer in Wireless Planning & Coordination Wing of Department of Telecommunications (DOT), Ministry of Communications & IT, Government of India. In DOT, he is associated with spectrum management activities, including spectrum planning and engineering and policy regarding regulatory affairs for new technologies and related research & development activities and ITU-R related matters.

Dr. Tripathi has also been associated with the implementation of a very prestigious World Bank Project on National Radio Spectrum Management and Monitoring System (NRSMMS). This project includes automation of Spectrum Management processes and design, supply, installation/commissioning of HF/VHF/UHF fixed monitoring stations;

V/UHF mobile monitoring stations; LAN/WAN communications network, etc. His areas of interest include Radio Regulatory affairs for new technologies and cognitive radio. He has also worked as a research fellow in Department of Electronics, University of Tor Vergata, Rome, Italy. Presently he is pursuing his Ph.D. on Cognitive Radio from Aalborg University, Aalborg, Denmark under the supervision of Professor Ramjee Prasad.

Ramjee Prasad (R) is a distinguished educator and researcher in the field of wireless information and multimedia communications. Since June 1999, Professor Prasad has been with Aalborg University (Denmark), where currently he is Director of Center for Teleinfrastruktur (CTIF, www.ctif.aau.dk), and holds the chair of wireless information and multimedia communications. He is coordinator of European Commission Sixth Framework Integrated Project MAGNET (My personal Adaptive Global NET) Beyond. He was involved in the European ACTS project FRAMES (Future Radio Wideband Multiple Access Systems) as a Delft University of Technology (the Netherlands) project leader. He is a project leader of several international, industrially funded projects. He has published over 500 technical papers, contributed to several books, and has authored, coauthored, and edited over 30 books. He has supervised over 50 PhDs and 15 PhDs are at the moment working with him. He has served as a member of the advisory and program committees of several IEEE international conferences. In addition, Professor Prasad is the coordinating editor and editor-in-chief of the Springer International Journal on *Wireless Personal Communications* and a member of the editorial board of other international journals. Professor Prasad is also the founding chairman of the European Center of Excellence in Telecommunications, known as HERMES, and now he is the Honorary Chair. He has received several international awards; the latest being the "Telenor Nordic 2005 Research Prize". He is a fellow of IET, a fellow of IETE, a senior member of IEEE, a member of The Netherlands Electronics and Radio Society (NERG), and a member of IDA (Engineering Society in Denmark). Professor Prasad is advisor to several multinational companies. In November 2010, Ramjee Prasad received knighthood from the Queen of Denmark, the title conferred on him is Riddere af Dannebrog.

Green by ICT

Basavaraj Hooli

MphasiS Ltd., CC2, Magarapatta, Pune 411028, India;
e-mail: basavaraj.hooli@mphasis.com

Received 13 September 2011; Accepted: 28 September 2011

Abstract

Information and Communication Technology (ICT) consumes energy. Though ICT is responsible for 2% of global carbon emission, it helps in conserving the energy. Conventionally, it has done so by optimizing the performance of energy-using systems and processes in industry and commerce. In the near future, ICT will play a critical role in supporting the necessary paradigm shifts in the human behaviour through better understanding of the ecological impact by the various industry sectors by providing the necessary data and the awareness. Through Life Cycle Assessment tools, ICT will help in optimizing the use of energy. Within the energy sector, ICT will help towards more sustainable electricity generation. With the advent of 'smart' technology from the field of ubiquitous computing, further ways of reducing growing levels of domestic energy consumption are now emerging. As per some reports Applications of ICT could enable emissions reductions of 15% of business-as-usual emissions. ICT will be instrumental in helping to develop new, climate-friendly technologies that can help economy's growth sustain ably and reduce emissions in the years ahead. This paper is towards giving more understanding of the Life Cycle Assessment and how it could become a key factor in reducing the rate of climate change.

Keywords: life cycle assessment, energy management, energy convergence, ecological intelligence.

Journal of Green Engineering, Vol. 2, 45–54.

1 Introduction

Climate change is no longer a topic of scientific debate now. It is a real concern we face today. Carbon emission is the centre stage and the focal point of analysts and accountants and is already a major factor that will determine the economy of various countries. The reduction of consumption and energy efficiency has become the focus in the balance sheets of various companies all around the world today. Al Gore, Former Vice President of United States of America, in his Oscar winning documentary – 'Inconvenient Truth' has warned about the perils of Global Warming which include rising sea levels, unpredictable weather patterns, changing seasons, depleting ozone layers, rising CHGs and green house effect. All this is happening in the last 14 years with 2011 also seeing hurricane Irene, highest temperature of greater than 100 degrees experienced by some of the eastern states of USA.

In view of rising temperatures and global warming, environmental sustainability has become more important in recent years. It is all about managing the natural resources in a better and more efficient way. This will help arresting the rising energy costs. A growing number of large infrastructure systems and processes have been optimized to consume less power. With its general potential for large-scale simulation, optimization, and real-time control, ICT plays a leading role here. In a business context, ICT is also being used to make better decisions relating to resource and energy consumption – examples include optimizing production and supply chain processes [1], and developing environmental information systems [1]. Investments in energy-saving technologies often also pay off financially, particularly when energy costs are rising.

ICT has an important indirect impact on the overall use of natural resources and energy, the total energy consumption of ICT itself is difficult to estimate. Studies vary depending on the definition of ICT, the methodology used to generate the estimates, and the proportion of a device's energy consumption that is attributed to ICT [1]. Irrespective of the data, the percentage share of total electricity consumption by the ICT sector is quite significant and warrants attention and calls for appropriate measures to be taken. Indeed, quite some effort has already been undertaken to address this issue, striving for low-energy ICT systems. The drivers are manifold and include several incentives over and above environmental considerations ('green ICT'), such as the cost of running large data centres, challenges related to heat dissipation from processors, and the working lifetime of battery-operated devices.

High hopes rest upon ICT to reduce resource and energy consumption in other economic sectors, and thus mitigate global warming. For example, ICT could help to improve the energy efficiency of established processes (i.e., increasing the ratio of a relevant target variable such as productivity or convenience to energy consumption), or it might be used to develop new concepts to generate, allocate, distribute, share, and use energy in a resource-efficient and environmentally-friendly way.

There are substantial inefficiencies in the technology, business and user behaviours that can be readily addressed with ICT. This paper is about bringing out the inefficiencies and the tools with the aid of ICT to address them in the context of environment impact and also discuss the Life Cycle Assessment in regard to changing of the buying patterns that consider the environmental effect (eco friendly procurement).

2 Energy Is Just Another Resource That Needs Managing

Any energy from its source of generation to consumption will have losses in its path. Not all the energy that is generated will be put into the productive usage. Figure 1 depicts the percentage of energy actually put into use in a typical IT scenario.

Figure 1 shows that there is only a small percentage of energy that is put into the real use while the majority does not do the real work. Most of the energy is lost in the form of heat. Because of the heat dissipation, there additional work of maintaining the cooling systems. This is the non productive work that consumes more energy. This is where there is an opportunity for improving the efficiency.

2.1 Smart Grid

Let us take another example of electric grids, generation, transmission and distribution; there is a transmission loss of close to 30%. Electric grids are another example to show the extent of losses from generation to consumption. It is actually only a small percentage of the electricity generated that does the productive work. This calls for some mechanism to manage the losses. ICT plays a vital role in managing this. Figure 2 is schematic of smart grids that will help reducing the losses with smart technology.

Smart grid is a generic label for the application of computer intelligence and networking abilities to a dumb electricity distribution system. Smart grid initiatives seek to improve operations, maintenance and planning by making

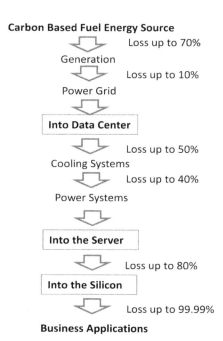

Figure 1 Percentage of energy put into actual use. (Source: Gartner)

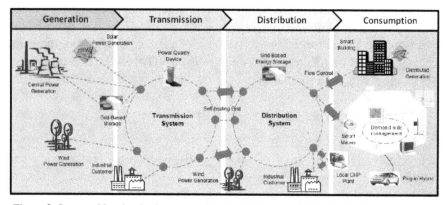

Figure 2 Smart grid technologies across the electricity sector value chain. (Source: OECD)

sure that each component of the electric grid can both 'talk' and 'listen'. Another major component of smart grid technology is automation. Through the use of ICT and management of energy losses, it is possible to increase its efficiency close to 47% [3].

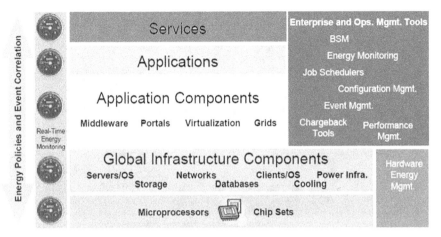

Figure 3 Integrated ICT energy management architecture. (Source: Gartner)

2.2 Energy Management Architecture

The best way of managing the energy is to have an energy monitoring system which serves as a feedback for corrective actions to be taken. It is essential to have some kind of energy policies. Figure 3 is Gartner's proposal for the dynamic, integrated ICT energy management architecture.

3 Energy Convergence

In order to manage the energy as an important resource, one has to look at it in a more holistic way than looking at each industry segment in isolation. This brings us to the concept of Convergence with Energy or Energy convergence. Smart grids are the convergence of Electric Network with ICT. By combining home automation and automobiles along with different energy sources with ICT, we can have a more holistic view of the its usage and thereby enable us to optimally manage the energy usage. Figure 4 depicts the next wave of convergence with energy.

The convergence should also be looked at from global perspective in terms of how the different countries can collaborate in achieving the convergence. The learning's from the Network Convergence in Telecom networks can be used to achieve this.

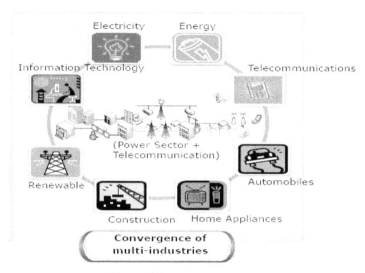

Figure 4 Energy convergence.

4 Adopting Ecological Intelligence

It is not sufficient to just look at the products that consume less power or the products that are bio-de gradable in order to protect the environment. It is important to know the process by which these products have been produced including the raw material and how it has impacted the environment in the process of getting into the product shape. The term 'Ecological Intelligence' is coined by Daniel Goleman to describe a new kind of math for the environmentally concerned, one that answers those everyday eco-conundrums like, which is better: a reusable stainless steel water bottle, or those throwaway plastic ones?

The answers come from life cycle assessment (or LCA), the method used by industrial ecologists – a discipline that blends industrial engineering and chemistry with environmental science and biology – to assess how man-made systems impact natural ones. LCAs tells us that buying food in one store that has been shipped in bulk leaves a smaller carbon footprint than driving around town to the local bakery, farmer's market, and dairy. Or that the better wine choice for those living east of Columbus, Ohio, is a French Bordeaux, and for those to the west it is the Napa Valley.

Let us take a specific example of whether to use a paper bag or a plastic. Figure 5 shows the life cycle for the paper grocery sack against the polyethylene grocery sack.

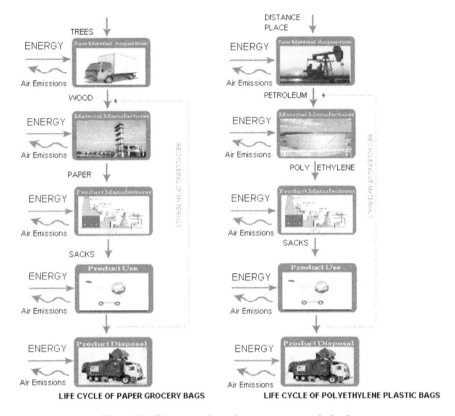

Figure 5 LCA comparisons between paper and plastic.

Figure 6 reveals more about the impact the two had on the environment in the process of creating the end product (sack).

Figures 5 and 6 clearly show the fact that paper sack has a more harmful effect on the environment compared to the plastic sack. Ecological intelligence is about understanding this. We now have products that come with a tag about how energy efficient they are with respect to energy consumption. Soon we will have the products that come with the tag about the impact they had on the environment while getting into their shape. This would change buyers decisions and might get a whole new way of producing and marketing.

Pollutant	Plastic Sacks		Paper Sacks	
	0% recycling	100% recycling	0% recycling	100% recycling
Particulates	0.8	0.8	24.5	2.8
Nitrogen Oxide	2.1	1.7	9.2	8.0
Hydrocarbons	5.8	3.2	4.9	3.9
Sulfur dioxides	2.6	2.7	13.6	10.6
Carbon monoxides	0.7	0.6	7.0	6.5
Aldehydes	0.0	0.0	0.1	0.1
Other Organics	0.0	0.0	0.3	0.2
Odorous sulfur	0.0	0.0	4.5	0.0

Life Cycle Stages	Air Emission (oz/sack)		Energy Consumption (Btu/sack)	
	Paper	Plastic	Paper	Plastic
Material processing + product manufacture + product Use	0.0516	0.0146	905	454
Raw materials acquisition + product disposal	0.0510	0.0045	724	185

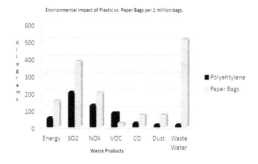

Figure 6 Environmental impact of paper sack against plastic sack.

5 Life Cycle Assessment (LCA)

What we think of as 'green' turns out to be less so (and sometimes more so) than we assume, when viewed through the lens of life cycle assessment or LCA, a method used by industrial ecologists – a discipline that blends industrial engineering and chemistry with environmental science and biology – to assess how manmade systems impact natural ones. LCAs, for example, yield a fine-grained analysis of the environmental and health impacts of a stainless steel bottle from the extraction or concoction of its ingredients and its manufacture, through distribution, use and final disposal. We are all concerned about carbon footprints these days. But for stainless steel the main concerns in addition to climate change are releases into the environment of particulates and human toxins, depletion of fossil fuels and natural resources, and eco-toxicity.

The 21st century has inherited from the 20th (and sometimes the 19th) a legacy of manufacturing processes and a palette of industrial chemicals that were developed in a more innocent age, when no one knew – or cared that much – about the impacts of industry on nature. Today LCA, among other methods, makes these impacts vividly clear. This end of innocence presents a vast entrepreneurial opportunity: we need to re-invent everything, starting with the most basic methods of commerce and industry.

5.1 LCA Definition

Life Cycle Assessment (LCA) is a method developed to evaluate the mass balance of inputs and outputs of systems and to organize and convert those inputs and outputs into environmental themes or categories relative to resource use, human health and ecological areas. The quantification of inputs and outputs of a system is called Life Cycle Inventory (LCI). At this stage, all emissions are reported on a volume or mass basis (e.g., kg of CO_2, kg of cadmium, cubic meter of solid waste). Life Cycle Impact Assessment (LCIA) converts these flows into simpler indicators.

5.2 ISO 14040: 2006

ISO 14040:2006 describes the principles and framework for life cycle assessment (LCA) including: definition of the goal and scope of the LCA, the life cycle inventory analysis (LCI) phase, the life cycle impact assessment (LCIA) phase, the life cycle interpretation phase, reporting and critical review of the LCA, limitations of the LCA, the relationship between the LCA phases, and conditions for use of value choices and optional elements.

ISO 14040:2006 covers life cycle assessment (LCA) studies and life cycle inventory (LCI) studies. It does not describe the LCA technique in detail, nor does it specify methodologies for the individual phases of the LCA.

This series of standards allows making reliable and reusable Life Cycle Assessments. It is essential when making an LCA to refer to these standards so that the job would be acknowledged.

6 Conclusions

Green is a process not a status. We need to think of 'green' as a verb not as an adjective. This kind of shift in our mindset needs to occur if we wish to start looking at greening the earth or reducing the environmental impact by the industry. Having awareness about the Ecological Intelligence would help and the Industries need to follow LCA.

ICT, when used in a 'smart' way, will significantly help to reduce our society's demand for carbon-based energy, while at the same time offering interesting business opportunities for industry and guaranteeing a desirable lifestyle for its citizens.

References

[1] Friedemann Mattern, Thorsten Staake, and Markus Weiss. ICT for Green – How Computers Can Help Us to Conserve Energy, www.smart2020.org.
[2] Daniel Goleman. *Ecological Intelligence*. Penguin Books, 2009.
[3] Gyu Myoung Lee. Benefits and Barriers to Smart Grid – The Korean Example. Presented at OECD Technology Foresight Forum, Smart ICTs and Green Growth, Paris, 29 September 2010.
[4] ISO 14040:2006: ISO Standards.
[5] David Cohen. *Carbon Management and ICT*. Kirklees Council.
[6] Simon Mingay. *Green IT : A New Industry Shock Wave*. Gartner, 2007.
[7] SMART 2020: Enabling the Low Carbon Economy in the Information Age.

Biography

Basavaraj Hooli completed his M.Tech. in Computer Science and Engineering from IIT Bombay. A strong technology professional and a Telecom domain specialist with 25 years of experience out of which last 12 years have been in the Telecom Domain. His expertise are in solution design, capability building, innovation and delivering large programs to international clients. With the skills in enterprise architecture consulting and leadership development, He brings along unique combination of delivery skills with domain, technology and leadership building. He is an active member and vice president of Indian Telecom Standards body (www.gisfi.org) where he is working in the SeON (Service Oriented Networks) study group. He also leads the Mobility and Telco SiG of SRII in India

In his 25 years in the IT industry, he has played multiple roles including those of CTO & Vice President and with a major career profile in delivering large programs to international clients and capability building. He is currently with MphasiS limited, Pune (India) as Head – Enterprise Mobility Practice where he is involved in building Enterprise Mobile Applications.

Energy-Efficiency of Cooperative Sensing Schemes in Ad Hoc WLAN Cognitive Radios

Reshma Syeda and Vinod Namboodiri

Department of Electrical Engineering & Computer Science,
Wichita State University, 1845 Fairmount St., Wichita, KS 67260, USA;
e-mail: {rssyeda, vinod.namboodiri}@wichita.edu

Received 13 September; Accepted: 28 September

Abstract

In cognitive radio networks, the secondary users need to coordinate among themselves to reap the benefits of cooperative spectrum sensing. In this paper, we study and analyze the energy efficiency of two generic cooperative sensing schemes in an ad hoc WLAN backdrop – distributed cooperative sensing scheme and centralized cluster based cooperative sensing scheme. We further propose corresponding enhanced and adaptive versions of these two schemes where only an α fraction of nodes sense in each sensing cycle, as opposed to all the nodes in the network. Using an analytical energy model for sensing, we quantify the energy costs of each of these schemes and perform a comparative numerical analysis to demonstrate the amount of energy savings of the proposed cooperative schemes over their generic counterparts and non-cooperative schemes.

Keywords: cognitive radio, cooperative sensing, energy efficiency, WLAN.

1 Introduction

The world has witnessed a great deal of change this decade when it comes to wireless technologies. Be it Wi-Fi, WiMAX, WSNs or any other sub technology belonging to one of these areas, these technologies have permeated so deep into our lives that it is hard to imagine our lifestyles without them. However, with demand comes scarcity. The spectrum allocated to these technologies is greatly limited and hence the scarcity which emphasizes the great need to deal with and overcome this issue. Figures 1 and 2 show the spectrum measurements taken by FCC and the shared spectrum company respectively. It is clearly noticeable that only a few frequency bands are in use while about 70% of the remaining spectrum (mainly belonging to legacy radio technologies) remains unused for longer periods of time [1, 2]. This is where the opportunistic spectrum access (OSA) comes into picture. Through OSA, users can utilize the spectrum currently being unused especially when it comes to licensed spectrum of legacy technologies. One example is the TV spectrum. However, for a radio to use the spectrum opportunistically it should be aware and intelligent enough to look out for such vacant spectrum bands. Hence there is a great need to build better and intelligent radios and this is where the phrase 'cognitive radio' comes from. Cognition is the psychological result of perception and reasoning. This term was first coined by Mitola [3] in his PhD research work, though lately this has become synonymous with the term Dynamic Spectrum Access (DSA) in the sense that the goal of DSA/OSA is achieved through the cognition of the radio.

Cognitive Radios (CRs) opportunistically cash in on the licensed spectrum allocated to rightful owners that is not being used in time, frequency, space and code dimensions of a signal at a given instant (also called spectral opportunities) in order to make their communications efficient in terms of throughput, energy and delay metrics. Studies have shown that 90% of the time, the valuable licensed spectrum was found to be unoccupied [1]. However, on the contrary, with the advent of portable gadgets, the unlicensed spectrum for technologies like Wi-Fi is being crowded most of the times.

Hence, dealing with Wi-Fi crowding phenomenon is critically important for sustainable wireless computing for our future generations. One of the most recent endeavors in this direction was made by FCC which approved and reallocated the use of Television White Spaces (TVWS) for Wi-Fi. Such renovated Wi-Fi technology capable of using TVWS via cognition was renamed as White-Fi (IEEE standard 802.11af), sometimes also called 'Wi-Fi on Steroids'. TV channels 2–52 have been opened up for unlicensed usage by the general public. Though the FCC recently has agreed to ditch the spectrum sensing requirement and instead encourage the use of online databases for spectrum vacancy [22, 23], it would still be an undeniable component when considering an 'on the fly' ad hoc Wi-Fi network that does not have access to these online databases.

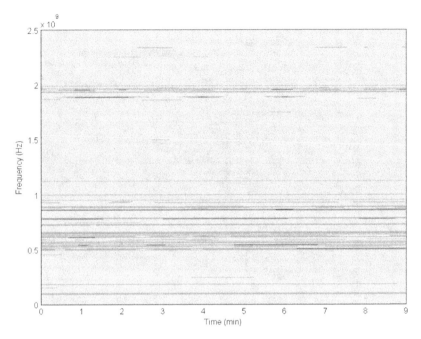

Figure 1 FCC spectrum measurements.

In the field of CR technology, the rightful users of the licensed spectrum are termed the Primary Users (PUs) where as the other CR users trying to use this spectrum opportunistically are the Secondary Users (SUs). The SUs, before dynamically accessing this licensed spectrum should make sure that it is not being used by any PU in their local vicinity so as to avoid interference to the PUs. The key component to achieve this is the sensing of the spectrum with high reliability.

As the transmitter based sensing techniques like energy detection [4, 5], matched filtering [6], cyclostationary [7] feature detection rely solely on the PU signal detection, there is a high chance for the cognitive user to be blinded by fading, shadowing and interference which might further degrade the accuracy of these techniques. The affects of these degradations have been studied in [8]. To overcome these blinding phenomena, cooperative sensing has been found to be far superior to just local/non-cooperative sensing as it solves the hidden node problem in addition to the others mentioned.

However, there is limited literature that looks at the energy cost aspect of the cognitive radio technology. One work that does and is our point of

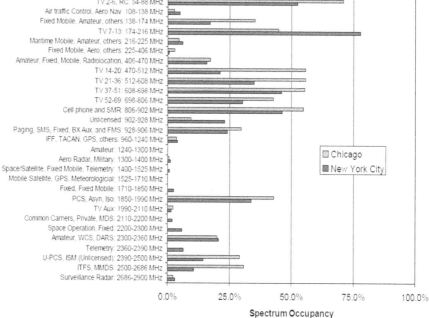

Figure 2 Spectrum measurements in New York City and Chicago conducted by Shared Spectrum, 2005.

interest is [9] which looks at the positive and negative impact of CR MAC layer sensing in terms of energy. However, this work does not look at the energy costs of cooperative sensing; and the techniques (optimal scan and greedy scan schemes) proposed here are non-cooperative sensing schemes. Our work in this paper is a subsequence to that with a goal to minimize the energy spent in spectrum sensing for each node and the network as a whole through cooperative sensing schemes. The following are the specific contributions made in this paper:

- We developed an energy model to study and quantify the energy costs of a broader class of existing generic cooperative MAC layer sensing schemes – one based on a distributed architecture and one based on a centralized architecture.

- We proposed corresponding new α-schemes – α-distributed and α-centralized where only a fraction α of the nodes scan as opposed to all the nodes in the generic distributed and centralized schemes.
- We numerically evaluated and compared the energy consumption costs of the generic distributed and centralized schemes against the proposed α-distributed and α-centralized schemes.
- We studied optimal values of α and number of nodes in the network N.
- We made a conclusive energy comparison study of non-cooperative sensing schemes and cooperative schemes.

The rest of the paper is organized as follows: related work is discussed in Section 2; an overview of the current sensing schemes and the proposed α-schemes is given in Section 3. In Section 4 we discuss the system model based on which further energy consumption analysis equations are developed in Section 5 and energy savings analysis done in Section 6. Numerical evaluations of these equations are done in Section 7 followed by an interpretation of their significance.

2 Related Work

This section gives a short overview of the prior work done in cognitive network cooperative sensing schemes with more emphasis placed on the two well known CR cooperative sensing implementations – distributed and centralized cluster based schemes. In a distributed cooperative sensing scheme, the SUs share the sensed information among themselves and make individual decisions. The advantage here is that there is no need for a common receiver infrastructure and high bandwidths [10]. Distributed collaboration schemes are discussed in [11]. In [12, 13] relay based cooperation are discussed where a few SUs act as relays to other SUs. In [13], the Amplify and Relay (AR) and Detect and Relay (DR) schemes are proposed for sensor networks.

In a centralized cooperative sensing system model, there is a common receiver which collects all the sensing information done by the SUs (CRs). Our interest is mainly on the cluster based schemes where the SUs are grouped into clusters or teams for collaboration; the reason being that to design an energy efficient cooperative sensing scheme, grouping would be a key component to cash in on the team collaboration instead of putting the burden of sensing the huge spectrum on each SU [14]. By grouping the SUs into clusters and selecting the most favourable SU in every cluster to report to the common receiver, the sensing performance can be greatly enhanced [15].

In [16] a study is carried out on the optimal number of clusters required to minimize the communication overhead without loss in the detection performance. In [17], two level hierarchical cluster based architecture is proposed where the low level collaboration is among the SUs within a cluster and high level collaboration is among the cluster heads chosen for each cluster. Other grouping techniques are studied in [18–21].

Although many variations of cooperative sensing schemes exist, our objective is to study the amount of energy consumption in both these categories. Also we propose the improved versions of both the generic distributed and centralized scheme and demonstrate the relative energy savings through evaluations.

Most of the work done till to date on cooperative sensing in CR networks mainly focus on increasing the throughput and spectrum sensing efficiency/accuracy. Not much has been done on analyzing how energy efficient these schemes are.

Also as there is no consensus over which specific scanning scheme performs the best, we chose to look at a generic class of distributed and centralized schemes and apply our energy model to evaluate their energy consumption. The following section gives a brief overview of the existing sensing schemes and the proposed α-schemes.

3 Overview of Sensing Schemes

Spectrum sensing is a key critical component in the cognitive radio technology since the ability of cognition is achieved through this spectrum sensing functionality of the CR. These spectrum sensing schemes can be roughly classified into two categories.

3.1 Non-Cooperative Sensing

Non-cooperative sensing schemes also called as local sensing schemes require each node in the network to sense the spectrum for free channels individually. These nodes do not share the scanned information with their neighbours and hence no reporting is involved in a non-cooperative sensing cycle. The non-cooperative sensing we use as reference in our work is the optimal scan scheme from [9]. In this optimal scan scheme, every node has to scan all the channels before choosing the optimal channel among them.

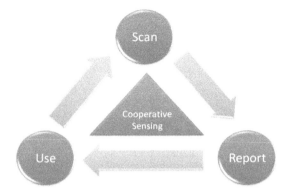

Figure 3 Cooperative sensing cycle.

3.2 Cooperative Sensing

In cooperative sensing schemes, all the nodes in the network sense/scan the spectrum and share this information with all the neighbouring nodes in the reporting phase (see Figure 3). This process reduces the CR blinding due to interference, fading and hence increases the probability of PU detection. To be precise, the collaboration of SUs can either be used to increase the number of channels scanned or improve the detection probabilities by having multiple nodes scan a single channel. In this paper, we look at more of a parallel cooperative sensing [24] where all the nodes are designated different channels to be scanned. Each node individually scans the designated channels in parallel (concurrently) and then convey this information through its sensing reports (SR).

Each sensing cycle (SC) has a scanning period (SP) and a reporting period (RP). Based on how the reporting/sharing is accomplished in the reporting period, cooperative sensing can be categorized into mainly two broad classes of architectures – distributed and centralized. The generic distributed sensing scheme we refer in this work belongs to the distributed architecture and is hereafter referred to as 'distributed sensing scheme' and the generic centralized cluster based scheme belongs to the centralized architecture which is hereafter referred to as the 'centralized cluster based scheme'.

3.2.1 Distributed Sensing Scheme

In the distributed sensing scheme as shown in Figure 4, each node scans its share of channels during the SP and shares this information with all its neighbors in the RP.

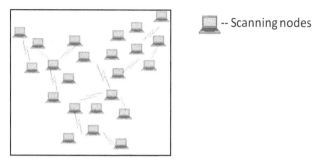

Figure 4 Distributed scheme.

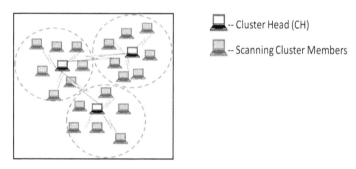

Figure 5 Centralized scheme.

3.2.2 Centralized Cluster Based Sensing Scheme

In the centralized cluster based scheme as shown in Figure 5, the whole network of nodes can be divided into clusters (based on some higher layer protocol). Each cluster has a cluster head (CH) which does not carry out the scanning. Only the cluster members (CMs) in each cluster scan their share of the channels and convey this information to their respective CH. The CHs then share this information with the other remaining CHs in the network. There are two levels of communication happening here, one at the intra cluster level and the other at the inter cluster level between the CHs. At the end of the inter cluster level information exchange, all the nodes in the network have a global view of the channel information for the whole network (see Figure 5).

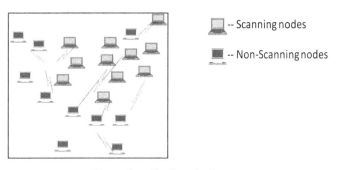

Figure 6 α-distributed scheme.

3.3 Proposed α-Sensing Schemes

Next, we propose the α-sensing schemes to make the conventional schemes more energy efficient. In the α-sensing schemes only a fraction α of nodes share the burden of scanning the channels in each sensing cycle. This is a form of load sharing which saves energy for the other fraction of nodes in that sensing cycle and simultaneously the scanning of all the channels is collectively completed by the end of the sensing cycle. This fraction of nodes can be chosen based on their SNRs and PDRs (Probability Detection Ratios) to attain better spectrum sensing accuracies.

3.3.1 α-Distributed Sensing Scheme
In the α-distributed sensing scheme as shown in Figure 6, only an α fraction of nodes scan the channels in a given sensing cycle. However they still share this information with all their neighbouring nodes just similar to the generic distributed sensing scheme. This saves energy, as each node has to scan only an α percentage of the times on average, in any given number of sensing cycles. This subset of α nodes can be chosen based on a probabilistic random number generator. For every SP, each node, through a probabilistic method (random number generator) decides to participate in scanning if the generated value is less than the 'α' value. This way on an average each node in the network scans once in '$(1/\alpha)$' sensing cycles (see Figure 6).

3.3.2 α-Centralized Cluster Based Sensing Scheme
In this α-centralized sensing scheme as shown in Figure 7, instead of all the CMs in the cluster scanning for channels, only a fraction α of the CMs share the scanning responsibility and report this information to the CH. The CH in turn shares this information with other CHs similar to the centralized scheme.

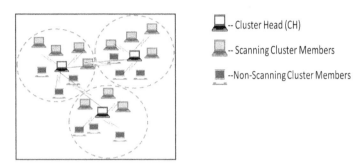

Figure 7 α-centralized scheme.

Once the CHs receive all the other cluster scan information, each CH shares a final report with its CMs. The fraction α of the CMs in each cluster is chosen by the CH.

Although another option of choosing a fraction α of the clusters instead of fraction of CMs from each cluster is possible, keeping in consideration the spatial diversity benefits of the clusters in the case of varying channel characteristics, it is better to have the scanning carried out in all the clusters for better sensing accuracies.

To further study these schemes, the system model and the analytical energy model are developed in the next section.

4 System Model

4.1 Basic Common Aspects of the Cooperative Sensing Model

We envision a crowded ad hoc WLAN scenario where all the nodes are connected in a clique network and hence are in the hearing range of each other. Each node has two transceivers/radios – one completely dedicated for the sensing and reporting purpose and the other radio for data transmission (see Figure 8). The radio for sensing and reporting shifts to the channel(s) that needs to be scanned during the SP and finally switches to the control channel for reporting purposes. The other physical radio for data transmission switches to the vacant channel over which it could transfer the data.

At the end of the SP, each node shares a sensing report with all the remaining nodes through a single broadcast packet regardless of the number of channels scanned. Since the nodes perform parallel scanning, at the end of the reporting period every node would have the spectrum map of all the channels. We do not presume the existence of a fusion center in this 'on

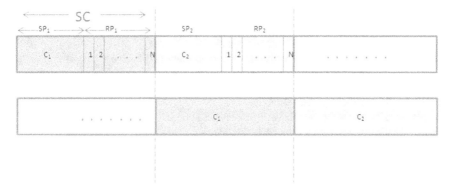

Figure 8 Time frame structures of scanning and reporting, data transmission respectively.

the fly' network for both the distributed and centralized architectures. In the distributed scheme, each node acts as a fusion centre for itself while in the centralized scheme the cluster head can take up this role for its cluster.

4.2 Orchestration

The total number of channels to be sensed 'C' by the network of 'N' nodes are decided prior to the start of SC. Since there is no reporting involved in the non-cooperative sensing scheme, each node scans all the C channels in the scanning period.

In the distributed cooperative sensing scheme, each node scans its share of designated channels in the SP. In the RP, it broadcasts this information to its $(N-1)$ neighbors and similarly decodes the $(N-1)$ reports it receives from its scanning neighbors. In the centralized scheme, each CM scans its share of designated channels and sends an SR to the CH. The CH after collecting all the SRs of its CMs, broadcasts an SR with this scan information of its cluster to all the other CHs in the network. Similarly, after receiving all the SRs from its peer CHs, each CH then sends a final consolidated SR having all the channel scan information to its CMs. Once these final SRs from the corresponding CHs are shared, all the CMs and CHs have a global view of all the channels scanned by the whole network.

4.3 Energy Model of Sensing Cycle

Energy consumed by each node per sensing cycle E_S is given by the sum of the total energy to scan all the assigned channel $E_{T_{\text{scan}}}$, the total energy to

Table 1 Definition of variables used [9].

Variable	Definition
P_{scan}	Power consumed to scan a channel (700 mW)
P_{sw}	Power consumed to switch once between channels (750 mW)
P_{tx}	Power consumed to transmit a packet (750 mW)
P_{rx}	Power consumed to receive a packet (750 mW)
T_{scan}	Time to scan a channel (50 ms)
T_{sw}	Time to switch once between channels (0.06 ms)
T_{data}	Time to transmit a Data packet (0.08 ms)
E_{scan}	Energy consumed to scan a channel $= P_{scan} T_{scan}$
E_{sw}	Energy consumed to switch once between channels $= P_{sw} T_{sw}$
E_{srt}	Energy consumed to transmit a Sensing Report (SR) $= P_{tx} T_{data}$
E_{srd}	Energy consumed to decode/receive a SR $= P_{rx} T_{data}$
C	Number of channels
N	Number of nodes in the network
N_S	Number of scanning nodes in the network
α	Fraction factor
K	Number of clusters into which the whole network of N nodes is divided/grouped
M_S	Number of scanning CMs

switch between these channels ETsw, the total energy to transmit/broadcast the SR(s) to the other nodes E_{T_x} and the total energy to receive the SRs from all the other nodes E_{R_x}.

$$E_S = E_{T_{scan}} + E_{T_{sw}} + E_{T_x} + E_{R_x}$$

Based on the above system and energy model developed, appropriate equations for energy consumption analysis are derived in the following section.

5 Energy Consumption Analysis of Sensing Schemes

5.1 Non-Cooperative Sensing Scheme

Since there is no reporting period in a non-cooperative sensing scheme, the energy consumed by each node is just the sum of the energy to scan the designated channels and the energy consumed to switch between those channels. Each node scans channels and hence has to switch times when hopping from one channel to another. Hence

$$E_{non-coop}^{S} = C E_{scan} + (C - 1) E_{sw}$$

where $E_{\text{non}-\text{coop}}^S$ is the energy consumed for each node during the scanning period. Total energy consumed by all the N nodes in the network to sense C channels in this non-cooperative sensing scheme is given by

$$E_{\text{non}-\text{coop}} = N E_{\text{non}-\text{coop}}^S$$
$$E_{\text{non}-\text{coop}} = N C E_{\text{scan}} + N(C-1)E_{\text{sw}} \qquad (1)$$

5.2 Distributed Sensing Scheme

In this generic scheme, each node scans $C/N (\geq 1)$ channels in each SP as long as $N > 1$. If $N > C$, not every node has to scan the channels. Hence the total energy for the whole network in the distributed scheme is given by the following generic equation:

$$E_{\text{dist}} = N_S E_{\text{dist}}^S + (N - N_S)E_{\text{dist}}^{N_S} \qquad (2)$$

where $N_S = \min(N, C)$ is the number of scanning nodes, E_{dist}^S is the energy consumed by the scanning node, $E_{\text{dist}}^{N_S}$ is the energy consumed by the non-scanning node. E_{dist}^S for a scanning node is the sum of energy to scan the designated (C/N_S) channels, switch in between those channels, transmit one SR with the channel scan information and receive $(N_S - 1)$ SRs from the other scanning nodes. $E_{\text{dist}}^{N_S}$ for a non-scanning node is the energy to decode all the SRs received from the scanning nodes.

$$E_{\text{dist}}^S = \left(\frac{C}{N_S}\right) E_{\text{scan}} + \left(\frac{C}{N_S} - 1\right) E_{\text{sw}} + E_{\text{srt}} + (N_S - 1)E_{\text{srd}} \qquad (3)$$

$$E_{\text{dist}}^{N_S} = N_S E_{\text{srd}} \qquad (4)$$

Substituting equations (3) and (4) in (2) gives rise to the following energy equation for the whole network of nodes of distributed scheme

$$E_{\text{dist}} = C E_{\text{scan}} + (C - N_S)E_{\text{sw}} + N_S E_{\text{srt}} + N_S(N - 1)E_{\text{srd}} \qquad (5)$$

Since $N_S = \min(N, C)$ we have the following two cases:

- If $N \leq C$, then

$$E_{\text{dist}} = C E_{\text{scan}} + (C - N)E_{\text{sw}} + N E_{\text{srt}} + (N^2 - N)E_{\text{srd}} \qquad (6)$$

- If $N > C$, then only C nodes are required to scan

$$E_{\text{dist}} = C E_{\text{scan}} + C E_{\text{srt}} + (NC - C)E_{\text{srd}} \qquad (7)$$

5.3 α-Distributed Sensing Scheme

In this scheme, for a chosen value of α ($0 < \alpha \leq 1$), only αN nodes perform the scanning while the remaining nodes do not scan for that SP. Hence for a given number of sensing cycles, the nodes in this scheme would have to scan only for α percentage of the cycles on an average while they can save on their energy for the remaining $(1 - \alpha)$ percentage of the cycles.

Practically, since the sensing nodes αN cannot be either less than 1 or for that matter greater than C, we arrive at the following bound for α:

$$\left(\frac{1}{N}\right) \leq \alpha \leq \min\left(\frac{C}{N}, 1\right) \tag{8}$$

Because of this α bound we can completely rule out the possibility of $\alpha N > C$ in this α-scheme.

Substituting $N_S = \alpha N$ in equations (2–4) gives the following energy equations for each of the scanning node and for the whole network respectively:

$$E^S_{\alpha-\text{dist}} = \left(\frac{C}{\alpha N}\right) E_{\text{scan}} + \left(\frac{C}{\alpha N} - 1\right) E_{\text{sw}} + E_{\text{srt}} + (\alpha N - 1) E_{\text{srd}} \tag{9}$$

$$E^S_{\alpha-\text{dist}} = C E_{\text{scan}} + (C - \alpha N) E_{\text{sw}} + \alpha N E_{\text{srt}} + \alpha (N^2 - N) E_{\text{srd}} \tag{10}$$

where $E^S_{\alpha-\text{dist}}$ is the energy consumed by the scanning node and $E_{\alpha-\text{dist}}$ is the energy consumed by the whole network of nodes.

5.4 Centralized Cluster Based Sensing Scheme

In this generic centralized scheme, the network of N nodes is divided into K clusters, each cluster having a group of $M+1$ nodes such that $N = K(M+1)$. Each cluster of $M + 1$ nodes thus has one cluster head (CH) and M cluster members (CMs). The CMs alone do the scanning and send their SRs to their respective CHs. Each CH then shares this information with the remaining CHs. A final SR is then broadcasted from the CH to its CMs.

Each cluster has to scan $(C/K)(\geq 1)$ channels and hence the energy consumed for each cluster per sensing cycle is

$$E^C_{\text{cent}} = E^{CH}_{\text{cent}} + M_S E^S_{\text{cent}} + (M - M_S) E^{NS}_{\text{cent}} \tag{11}$$

where $M_S = \min(M, C/K)$ is the number of scanning CMs, E^{CH}_{cent} is the energy consumed by the CH, E^S_{cent} is the energy consumed by the scanning CM, E^{NS}_{cent} is the energy consumed by the non-scanning CM.

Each CH transmits K SRs – one SR containing the scanned channel information of the cluster is unicast to each of the remaining $(K-1)$ CHs and one SR is broadcast back to the CMs after receiving all SRs from the $(K-1)$ CHs. Thus each CH has to decode all the M_S SRs from its CMs and $K-1$) SRs from the other CHs. For simplicity of evaluation, we consider a basic access mode of IEEE 802.11 [29] without RTS/CTS and ignore the energy for the ACK in the case of unicast transmission. For simplification, we further ignore the energy for the DIFS.

$$E_{\text{cent}}^{CH} = K E_{\text{srt}} + (M_S + (K-1) E_{\text{srd}} \tag{12}$$

Each CM transmits an SR to the CH after scanning $(C/K M_S)$ channels and decodes the final SR that it receives from its CH.

$$E_{\text{cent}}^{S} = \left(\frac{C}{K M_S}\right) E_{\text{scan}} + \left(\frac{C}{K M_S} - 1\right) E_{\text{sw}} + E_{\text{srt}} + E_{\text{srd}} \tag{13}$$

The energy consumed by the non-scanning CMs is

$$E_{\text{cent}}^{NS} = E_{\text{srd}} \tag{14}$$

$$E_{\text{cent}} = K E_{\text{cent}}^{C} \tag{15}$$

(15) Substituting equations (11–14) in (15) gives the energy equation for the whole network of nodes in the centralized scheme.

$$E_{\text{cent}} = C E_{\text{scan}} + (C - K M_S) E_{\text{sw}} + K (M_S + K) E_{\text{srt}}$$
$$+ K (M_S + M + K - 1) E_{\text{srd}} \tag{16}$$

Similar to the distributed scheme, if $M > (C/K)$ then not every CM has to scan in the cluster and hence we have the following two cases:

- If $M \le (C/K)$, then

$$E_{\text{cent}} = C E_{\text{scan}} + (C - K M) E_{\text{sw}} + K (M + K) E_{\text{srt}}$$
$$+ K (2M + K - 1) E_{\text{srd}} \tag{17}$$

- If $M > (C/K)$, then

$$E_{\text{cent}} = C E_{\text{scan}} + (C + K^2) E_{\text{srt}} + (C + K (M + K - 1)) E_{\text{srd}}$$
$$+ K (2M + K - 1) E_{\text{srd}} \tag{18}$$

5.5 α-Centralized Cluster Based Sensing Scheme

In this scheme, only αM CMs in each cluster do the scanning while the remaining $(M - \alpha M)$ CMs do not scan for that SP.

αM can neither be less than 1 and nor can it be greater than (C/K). (C/K) is the number of assigned channels for each cluster which would be the required number of scanning nodes too. Translating this to a mathematical bound gives the following:

$$\left(\frac{1}{M}\right) \leq \alpha \leq \min\left(\frac{C}{KM}, 1\right) \tag{19}$$

Because of this α bound we can completely rule out the possibility of $M_S > (C/K)$ in this scheme.

Substituting $M_S = \alpha M$ in equations (11–15) gives the following energy equation for the whole network of nodes in the α-centralized scheme:

$$E_{\alpha-\text{cent}} = CE_{\text{scan}} + (C - K\alpha M)E_{\text{sw}} + K(\alpha M + K)E_{\text{srt}}$$
$$+ K((1 + \alpha)M + (K - 1)E_{\text{srd}} \tag{20}$$

In the subsequent section, we analyze the energy savings and optimal values of α and N based on the above derived equations.

6 Energy Savings and Optimal Values

6.1 Energy Savings

Lemma 1. *Distributed cooperative sensing scheme is more energy-efficient than a non-cooperative scheme only when the number of nodes N is greater than 1 and the communication energy is less than*

$$\frac{(NC - C)E_{\text{scan}} + (NC - N - C + N_S)E_{\text{sw}}}{NN_S}$$

Proof. The distributed scheme saves energy over the non-cooperative scheme if and only if the total energy consumption for whole of network of nodes in the distributed scheme is less than the total energy consumption for the same network of nodes in the non-cooperative scheme. This is represented by the following relation:

$$E_{\text{dist}} \leq E_{\text{non-coop}} \tag{21}$$

Since communication is possible only when the network has more than one node, for the distributed scheme to be valid and equation (20) to hold, the following condition should be met:

$$N > 1$$

Solving equation (20) using equations (1) and (5) gives the following condition for communication energy:

$$E_{src} \leq \frac{(NC - C)E_{scan} + (NC - N - C + N_S)E_{sw}}{NN_S}$$

where $E_{src} = E_{srt} = E_{srd}$, $N_S = \min(N, C)$ for the distributed scheme and $N_S = \min(\alpha N, C)$ for the α-distributed scheme.

For ease of simplification, E_{srt}, E_{srd} in equation (5) are jointly denoted by E_{src} which is the communication energy in general. □

Lemma 2. *Centralized cluster based cooperative sensing scheme is energy-efficient than a non-cooperative scheme only when the number of clusters and the number of cluster members is at least 1 and the communication energy is less than*

$$\frac{(NC - C)E_{scan} + (NC - N - C + KM_S)E_{sw}}{K(2M_S + 2K + M - 1)}$$

Proof. The centralized scheme saves energy over the non-cooperative scheme if and only if the total energy consumption for whole of network of nodes in the centralized scheme is less than the total energy consumption for the same network of nodes in the non-cooperative scheme. This is represented by the following relation:

$$E_{cent} \leq E_{non-coop} \tag{22}$$

For a network to form a cluster, there should at least be one cluster and one cluster member in the cluster and hence we have

$$K \geq 1, \quad M \geq 1$$

Solving equation (21) using equations (1) and (16) gives the following condition for the communication energy:

$$E_{src} \leq \frac{(NC - C)E_{scan} + (NC - N - C + KM_S)E_{sw}}{K(2M_S + 2K + M - 1)}$$

where $E_{src} = E_{srt} = E_{srd}$, $M_S = \min(M, C/K)$ for the centralized scheme and $M_S = \min(\alpha M, C/K)$ for the α-centralized scheme. □

6.2 Optimal α Values for the α-Distributed Scheme

6.2.1 Optimal α for Maximum Energy Savings

The optimal α for given N is defined as the value of α where the energy savings of the α-distributed scheme over the distributed are the maximum. The energy savings can be looked at, from two different perspectives – the energy savings for the whole network of nodes and the energy savings per scanning node in the network. We first look at the optimal α for maximum energy savings considering the whole network of nodes over one sensing cycle paired with various constraints to form a set of optimization problems.

- *Optimization Problem 1 – Optimal α for a whole network of nodes*:

$$\text{Maximize } f(\alpha) = \left(\frac{E_{\text{dist}} - E_{\alpha-\text{dist}}}{E_{\text{dist}}} \right)$$

$$\text{such that } \left(\frac{1}{N} \right) \leq \alpha \leq \min \left(\frac{C}{N}, 1 \right)$$

The α value we consider optimal here, is the value of α where the α-distributed scheme shows the maximum energy savings over the distributed scheme considering the whole network of nodes for a given sensing cycle. $f(\alpha)$ is maximized at $\alpha = (1/N)$ which thus becomes the optimal α. However, considering the shadowing phenomenon, battery characteristics of the wireless nodes and most importantly the limited scanning and reporting periods, this value should be chosen with discretion in order to avoid poor spectral efficiencies and accuracies, shorter operating lifetimes respectively [28]. Hence a constraint to limit the sensing and reporting time in a given sensing cycle is needed as shown below in the next optimization problem.

- *Optimization Problem 2 – Optimal α for a whole network of nodes with time constraint*:

$$\text{Maximize } f(\alpha) = \left(\frac{E_{\text{dist}} - E_{\alpha-\text{dist}}}{E_{\text{dist}}} \right)$$

$$\text{such that } \left(\frac{1}{N} \right) \leq \alpha \leq \min \left(\frac{C}{N}, 1 \right) \text{ and } L \leq l$$

where L is the total time for the SC as defined below:

$$L = \left(\frac{C}{\alpha N} \right) T_{\text{scan}} + \left(\frac{C}{\alpha N} - 1 \right) T_{\text{sw}} + \alpha N T_{\text{data}} \tag{23}$$

In the evaluation section, we plot the optimal values where $f(\alpha)$ is maximized and the constraint $L \leq l$ ms is satisfied.

Also, for further study of the relative energy cost comparison of a scanning node in distributed scheme versus a scanning node in α-distributed scheme, we maximize the function $f(\alpha)$ with a scanning node energy constraint.

- *Optimization Problem 3 – Optimal α for a whole network of nodes with per scanning node energy constraint*:

$$\text{Maximize } f(\alpha) = \left(\frac{E_{\text{dist}} - E_{\alpha-\text{dist}}}{E_{\text{dist}}} \right)$$

$$\text{such that } \left(\frac{1}{N} \right) \leq \alpha \leq \min \left(\frac{C}{N}, 1 \right) \text{ and } g(\alpha) \geq 0$$

where

$$g(\alpha) = \left(\frac{E^S_{\text{dist}} - E^S_{\alpha-\text{dist}}}{E^S_{\text{dist}}} \right)$$

The $g(\alpha) \geq 0$ constraint was taken into account considering the fact that for a given sensing cycle, although the α-distributed scheme saves energy for the network of nodes N on the whole, it should not burden each scanning node with a very high number of channels to be scanned, causing the node to die quicker. This constraint makes sure that the energy of the scanning nodes in the α-distributed scheme is either less than or at least equal to the energy of scanning node in the distributed scheme. The optimal α with this constraint is always the upper bound of α given by $\min(C/N, 1)$. However if the constraint is relaxed to be less than zero, i.e., $g(\alpha) \leq 0$, the optimal would move to the lower bound which is $(1/n)$. $g(\alpha)$ thus helps to explain the fact that the per scanning node energy cost of α-distributed scheme versus that of the distributed over one sensing cycle is always higher except at $\min(C/N, 1)$ where it equals the distributed. In the next optimization problem, we show that the energy savings over a cumulative n sensing cycle period are however positive.

- *Optimization Problem 4 – Optimal α for maximum energy savings over n sensing cycle period*:

$$\text{Maximize } f(\alpha) = \left(\frac{E_{\text{dist}} - E_{\alpha-\text{dist}}}{E_{\text{dist}}} \right)$$

$$\text{such that } \left(\frac{1}{N}\right) \le \alpha \le \min\left(\frac{C}{N}, 1\right) \text{ and } h(\alpha) \ge 0$$

where

$$h(\alpha) = \left(\frac{\min\left(\frac{C}{N}, 1\right) E_{\text{dist}} S - (\alpha E^S_{\alpha-\text{dist}})}{\min\left(\frac{C}{N}, 1\right) E^S_{\text{dist}}}\right)$$

The constraint $h(\alpha)$ defines that, for a given n sensing cycle period each scanning node in the distributed scheme would have to scan $\min(C/N, 1) \times n$ times on an average while the scanning node in the α-distributed scheme would have to scan only for $\alpha \times n$ times on average. With this new constraint, the optimal α value is still $(1/N)$. However, the numerical evaluation results of $h(\alpha)$ show that the constraint itself results in positive values unlike the constraint $g(\alpha)$. This goes on to show that the α-distributed scheme saves energy from a scanning node's perspective as well as for the whole network over a given period of n sensing cycles and more noticeably at smaller α values.

6.2.2 Optimal *N* for Maximum Energy Savings

It is also interesting enough to analyze if there is an optimal N for a given α where the energy savings of the α-distributed over distributed are maximum. Hence we derive the optimal values of N for given fixed values of α by maximizing the function $F(N)$ where

$$F(N) = \left(\frac{E_{\text{dist}} - E_{\alpha-\text{dist}}}{E_{\text{dist}}}\right)$$

and solving it for maximization shows that it is maximized at

$$N = \max\left(\frac{-E_{\text{scan}} + \sqrt{E^2_{\text{scan}} + E_{\text{sw}} E_{\text{scan}}} + \left(\frac{C}{\alpha}\right) E_{\text{src}} E_{\text{scan}} + \left(\frac{C}{\alpha}\right) E_{\text{sw}} E_{\text{src}}}{E_{\text{src}}}, C\right)$$

Similarly, the function

$$G(N) = \left(\frac{\min\left(\frac{C}{N}, 1\right) E^S_{\text{dist}} - (\alpha E^S_{\alpha-\text{dist}})}{\min\left(\frac{C}{N}, 1\right) E^S_{\text{dist}}}\right)$$

for highest magnitude of energy savings per scanning node over n sensing cycles is maximized at $N = C$. We plot the values showing the trend of optimal N over a varying range of a for the functions $F(N)$ and $G(N)$ separately in the next section.

The outcomes of all the above optimizations are completely dependent on α, which is the basis of the relation between distributed and α-distributed. Since this relation remains the same between centralized and α-centralized, the optimization results and hence the inferences are going to be similar. So we do not look at optimizations for the centralized schemes in this work.

7 Evaluation

We do a numerical evaluation for all the proposed generic equations and show the energy savings of the α-schemes over their counterparts. All the base values for E_{scan}, E_{sw}, E_{srt}, E_{srd} are calculated from equations and values specified in [9, table 1]. Following [25] where White-Fi has to scan at least about 50 TV channels and [26] where the notion of channels can just be sub bands obtained by dividing a given wide band, we believe $C = 100$ would be a suitable and practical value for the number of channels to be scanned. In [27] the authors show that the optimal sensing time for a SU to detect the PU with 90% probability is about 15 ms and in [28] the false alarm probability had a linear down trend as scan time was varied from 20 to 100 ms. So we infer that $T_{scan} = 50$ ms would be an appropriate value to achieve a good detection probability and low false alarm rates simultaneously. We evaluate the total energy consumed for each of the schemes by varying the range of number of nodes N and the fraction factor α.

7.1 Distributed vs. α-Distributed Scheme

Figure 9 shows the energy trends over a varying N for the distributed and α-distributed schemes. The lower the value of α, the lesser are the energy costs for the α-distributed scheme. These energy savings become more apparent for higher node densities. However at the point the energy cost of the α-distributed scheme equals the distributed scheme and hence the energy savings decrease from positive values to zero. This is due to the fact that the significance of the fraction factor α lies only in the range suggested in equation (6), further explaining the point that there is no reason to have scanning nodes greater than the required number, which would be the number of channels C for both the distributed and the α-distributed schemes. Hence our proposed α-distributed scheme holds significance as long as $\alpha N < C$.

Figure 10 shows that the average energy costs of a node for both distributed and α-distributed keep decreasing with increasing node densities. A closer analysis indicates that this is due to the reduction in the scanning en-

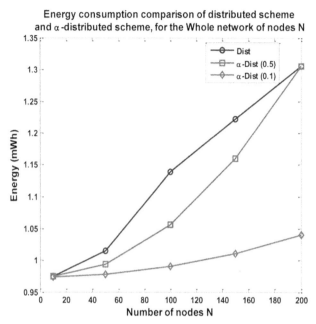

Figure 9 Total energy consumption of whole network of *N* nodes in distributed and α-distributed schemes.

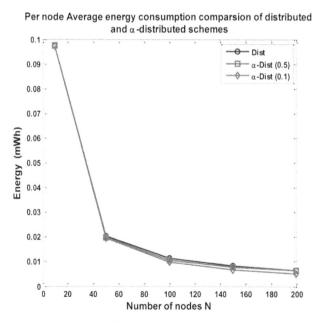

Figure 10 Average energy consumption of each node in distributed and α-distributed schemes.

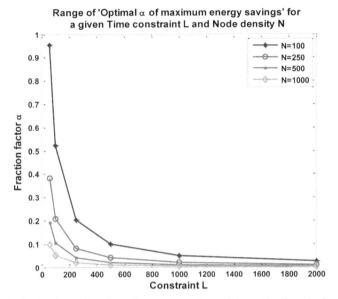

Figure 11 Optimal values of α where the energy savings of the α-distributed scheme over the distributed scheme are maximum, for a given N and L.

ergies; since with increasing node densities, the number of channels scanned on an average by each node keeps decreasing. Though the reporting energy increases on an average, this increase is greatly offset by the decrease in the scanning energy since $E_{scan} \gg E_{srt}$ (or) E_{srd}.

7.2 Optimal Values

The optimal α values for a given N where $f(\alpha)$ is maximized and the constraint of the sensing cycle time length L is satisfied are shown in Figure 11. It can be clearly noticed that the optimal α values decrease with increasing L. With higher L each node gets to scan more number of channels and so lesser scanning nodes are needed which results in a smaller α.

A further study of optimal values of N for a given α can be carried out using Figures 12 and 13. The function $F(N)$ has the highest magnitude of energy savings at various values of N for varying α until $\alpha = 0.5$, after which the optimal N stays at 100 (value of C). Optimal N for the function $G(N)$ is always at $N = C = 100$ regardless of the value of α. The energy savings for both and predictably go down with increasing α values.

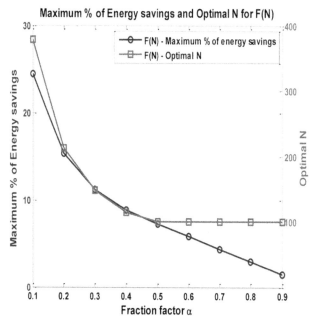

Figure 12 Percentage of energy savings and optimal N values where $F(N)$ is maximized.

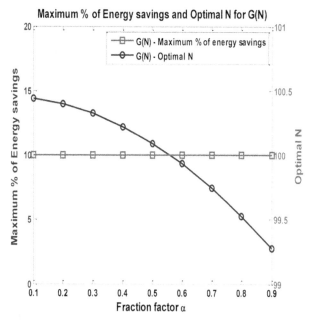

Figure 13 Percentage of energy savings and optimal N values where $G(N)$ is maximized.

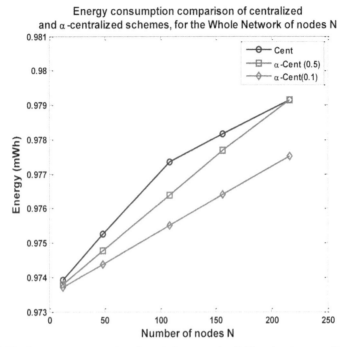

Figure 14 Total energy consumption for whole network of N nodes in centralized and α-centralized schemes.

7.3 Centralized vs. α-Centralized Schemes

Figure 14 shows the energy trends over a varying N for the centralized and α-centralized schemes. As expected, the centralized schemes in general have lower energy costs than the distributed schemes and the α-centralized schemes have lower energy costs over the centralized scheme.

The α-centralized schemes have lower energy costs with decreasing a and this can attributed to the lesser control overheads both for the CH and the CMs. Also, the energy increase with increasing N is more linear in the centralized schemes while this increase is inclined towards being exponential in the distributed schemes. This clearly shows that centralized schemes in general are more energy efficient and hence should be the first choice at higher N values. The values used in this plot were derived for $K = 1$. To gain further insight into the impact of K on energy consumption, we use Figure 15 which shows that a higher K results in higher energy overhead.

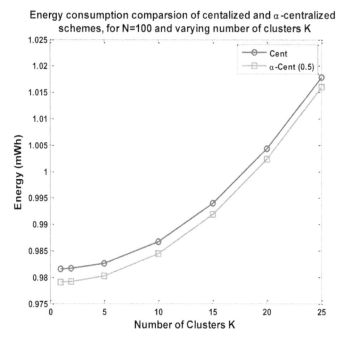

Figure 15 Impact of K on the total energy consumption for whole network of N nodes in centralized and α-centralized schemes.

7.4 Non-Cooperative vs. Cooperative Schemes

Cooperative schemes not only reduce the bandwidth requirements to convey the scanning information but also the energy consumed to scan and share this information. Figure 16 proves this claim and it can be noticed that a logarithmic scale was used to capture the wide variation of the energy values of non-cooperative schemes and the lower energy values of the cooperative schemes.

8 Conclusions

The energy model of sensing developed in this work gives a platform for an energy accountability, quantification and comparison of the non-cooperative sensing schemes and the generic cooperative sensing schemes – distributed and centralized along with our proposed new α-schemes. Our investigation on their energy costs shows that the cooperative schemes easily outperform the non-cooperative scheme and further the α-schemes are significantly energy

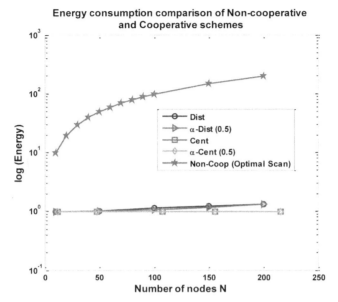

Figure 16 Energy consumption comparison of the non-cooperative and cooperative schemes.

efficient than the generic schemes. Optimal values for the fraction factor α and number of nodes N derived contribute to further useful insights on the relative energy savings.

References

[1] FCC. Et docket No. 03-322. Notice of Proposed Rule Making and Order, December 2003.
[2] Spectrum occupancy measurements performed by Shared Spectrum Company, http://www.sharedspectrum.com/papers/spectrum-reports, Chicage, Illinois, 2005.
[3] I. Mitola and G.Q. Maguire. Cognitive radio: Making software radios more personal. *IEEE Personal Commun.*, 6(4):13–18, 1999.
[4] D. Cabric, A. Tkachenko, and R. Brodersen. Spectrum sensing measurements of pilot, energy, and collaborative detection. In *Proceedings of IEEE Military Commun. Conference*, October 2006.
[5] D. Cabric, S. Mishra, and R. Brodersen. Implementation issues in spectrum sensing for cognitive radios. In *Proceedings of Asilomar Conference on Signals, Systems and Computers*, Vol. 1, 2004.
[6] R. Tandra and A. Sahai. Fundamental limits on detection in low SNR under noise uncertainty. In *Proceedings of IEEE International Conference on Wireless Networks, Communication and Mobile Computing*, 2005.

[7] M. Oner and F. Jondral. Cyclostationarity based air interface recognition for software radio systems. In *Proceedings of IEEE Radio and Wireless Conference*, September 2004.

[8] A. Ghasemi and E.S. Sousa. Asymptotic performance of collaborative spectrum sensing under correlated log-normal shadowing. *IEEE Commun. Lett.*, 11(1):34–36, 2007.

[9] V. Namboodiri. Are cognitive radios energy efficient? A study of the wireless LAN scenario. In *Proceedings of IEEE International Computing and Communications Conference*, 2009.

[10] Wenzhong Wang and Luyong Zhang. On the distributed cooperative spectrum sensing for cognitive radio. In *Proceedings of International Symposium on Communication and Information Technologies*, 2007.

[11] N. Ahmed, D. Hadaller, and S. Keshav. GUESS: Gossiping updates for efficient spectrum sensing. In *Proceedings International Workshop on Decentralized Resource Sharing in Mobile Computing and Networking*, 2006.

[12] J. Nicholas Laneman. Cooperative diversity in wireless networks: Efficient protocols and outage behavior. *IEEE Transactions on Information Theory*, 50(12), December 2004.

[13] Q. Chen and M. Motani. Cooperative spectrum sensing strategies for cognitive radio mesh networks. *IEEE Journal of Selected Topics in Signal Processing*, 2011.

[14] Chia-han Lee. Energy efficient techniques for cooperative spectrum sensing in cognitive radios. In *Proceedings IEEE Conference on Communications and Networking*, 2008.

[15] Chunhua Sun, Wei Zhang and K. Ben. Cluster-based cooperative spectrum sensing in cognitive radio systems. In *Proceedings IEEE International Conference on Communications*, 2007.

[16] Chen Guo and Tao Peng. Cooperative spectrum sensing with cluster-based architecture in cognitive radio networks. In *Proceedings Vehicular Technology Conference*, 2009.

[17] Bin Shen and Chengshi Zhao. User clusters based hierarchical cooperative spectrum sensing in cognitive radio networks. In *Proceedings IEEE International Conference on Cognitive Radio Oriented Wireless Networks and Communication*, 2009.

[18] Youmin Kim and Wonsop Kim. Group-based management for cooperative spectrum sensing in cognitive radio networks. *Proceedings International Conference on Advanced Communication Technology*, 2010.

[19] R. Akhtar, A. Rashdi, and A. Ghafoor. Grouping technique for cooperative spectrum sensing in cognitive radios. In *Proceedings International Workshop on Cognitive Radio and Advanced Spectrum Management*, 2009.

[20] Chunmei Qi Jun Wang. Weighted-clustering cooperative spectrum sensing in cognitive radio context. In *Proceedings International Conference on Communications and Mobile Computing*, 2009.

[21] Jiaqi Duan and Yong Li. A novel cooperative spectrum sensing scheme based on clustering and softened hard combination. In *International Conference on Wireless Communication, Networking and Information Security*, 2010.

[22] The Difference Engine: Bigger than Wi-Fi. http://www.economist.com/blogs/babbage/2010/09/white-space_wireless, 23 September 2010.

[23] Chloe Albanesius. FCC opens TV 'white spaces' for unlicensed super Wi-Fi, http://www.pcmag.com/article2/0,2817,2369580,00.asp, 23 September 2010.

[24] S. Xie, Y. Liu, Y. Zhang, and R. Yu. A parallel cooperative spectrum sensing in cognitive radio networks. *IEEE Transactions on Vehicular Technology*, 2010.

[25] L. Verma, Sim Daeyong, and S.S. Lee. Wireless networking in TV white space leveraging Wi-Fi. In *Proceedings of IEEE 14th International Symposium on Consumer Electronics*, 2010.

[26] A.R. Biswas, T.C. Aysal, S. Kandeepan, D. Kliazovich, and R. Piesiewicz. Cooperative shared spectrum sensing for dynamic cognitive radio networks. In *Proceedings IEEE International Conference*, 2009.

[27] Liang Ying-Chang, Zeng Yonghong, E.C.Y. Peh, and Hoang Anh Tuan. Sensing-throughput tradeoff for cognitive radio networks. *IEEE Transactions on Wireless Communications*, 2008.

[28] Kim Hyoil and K.G. Shin. Efficient discovery of spectrum opportunities with MAC-layer sensing in cognitive radio networks. *IEEE Transactions on Mobile Computing*, 2008.

[29] IEEE 802.11 Wireless Local Area Networks Standard – IEEE Standard for Information Technology. Telecommunications and information exchange between systems – Local and metropolitan area networks, http://standards.ieee.org/getieee802/download/802.11-2007.pdf.

Biographies

Reshma Syeda is currently a graduate student at Wichita State University, pursuing her M.S. degree in Electrical Engineering under the supervision of Professor Vinod Namboodiri. She has also worked as a graduate research assistant at the Cisco Technical Research Center of WSU. She received her B.Tech. degree in Electronics and Communications Engineering from Jawaharlal Nehru Technological University, India in 2007. Her research interests include cognitive radio networks and smart grids.

Vinod Namboodiri is currently an Assistant Professor at the Department of Electrical Engineering and Computer Science at Wichita State University, USA. He graduated with a Ph.D. in Electrical and Computer engineering from the University of Massachusetts Amherst in 2008. He has served or is currently serving on the technical program committees of IEEE GLOBECOM, IEEE ICC, IEEE IPCCC, and IEEE GREENCOM, and is an active reviewer for numerous journals and conferences in the mobile computing and green communications areas. His research interests include designing algorithms and protocols for energy-intelligent and sustainable computing, and designing an effective communication architecture for smart electric grids. In the past he has worked on designed MAC and routing protocols, and developing energy-efficient protocols and algorithms for different wireless technologies like Wireless LANs, RFID Systems, Wireless Sensor Networks, and Wireless Mesh Networks.

The Role of Wireless Sensor Networks for Green Gigabit Access Networks

V. Suraci

Department of Engineering, Università degli Studi e-Campus, Via Isimbardi 10, Novedrate (CO), 22060 Italy; e-mail: vincenzo.suraci@uniecampus.it

Received 17 September 2011; Accepted: 29 September 2011

Abstract

Actual home networks have become an heterogeneous environment in terms of technologies used and do not take into account any intelligent energy saving mechanism. In this paper we propose an energy saving strategy by integrating a Wireless Sensor Network (WSN) with a high speed, hybrid home network. The main objective is to demonstrate that a WSN can act as a dependable control plane, where low data rate control packets can flow even when the high speed home network is shut down. While the home network nodes or some of each node's network technologies can be deactivate, the WSN is always on and, due to the low data rate required to properly work, it consumes a very limited quantity of energy. This mutual interaction between the high speed home network and the WSN allows at the same time to achieve the convergence of heterogeneous communication technologies in the home environment and leads to a substantial reduction of the energy consumptions. Simulation results show that this strategy is effective in a multitude of scenarios and provides a tangible economic benefit.

Keywords: green, home network, gigabit access, future internet.

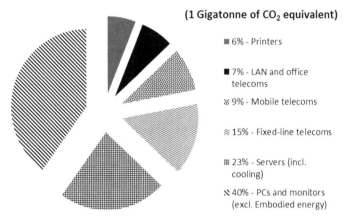

(1 Gigatonne of CO$_2$ equivalent)

■ 6% - Printers

■ 7% - LAN and office telecoms

≋ 9% - Mobile telecoms

≈ 15% - Fixed-line telecoms

⌗ 23% - Servers (incl. cooling)

⋉ 40% - PCs and monitors (excl. Embodied energy)

Figure 1 Green IT power consumption [21].

1 Introduction

The European countries are facing a hard period since the economic crisis coming from the US has passed the Ocean and has spread into the whole European economic and productive system. To avoid an endless crisis the EU has urgently approved a four years (2010–2013) European Economic Recovery Plan (EERP). The thrust of the EERP is to restore confidence of consumers and business. It is suggested to provide a demand stimulus of €200 billion [1]. The major instrument identified to apply the EERP strategy is the Public Private Partnership (PPP): an industry-driven RTDI initiatives tackling the major socio-economic challenges that look for maximizing EU industrial capabilities in order to allow their best exploitation for the EU industry of tomorrow, enhancing its competitiveness through high impact actions on research and innovation. In particular the PPP on the Future Internet initiative [2] identifies as the most important needs for the research and innovation green technologies and gigabit ICT for all the European citizens.

Recent publications [3–7] show that the ICT industry energy need is increasing with an exponential growth and it is about to exceed than the aviation industry. Thus the green ICT technologies are an emergent research field that needs pragmatic solutions [8]. While green ICT have been investigated in the context of core and access networks [9, 10], consistent improvements should be still done in the context of residential and office networks.

A study carried out by Gartner in 2007 (Figure 1) shows that the 7% of green ICT power consumption is due to home and office networks. It is a small portion of the whole ICT power consumption. So far systematic and integrated solutions to green this market sector do not exist. Some isolated initiatives have been taken by the manufacturers to improve the network elements efficiency and to make them more green. However the green ICT problem in home networks has never been faced with an integrated approach.

Today's homes are equipped with a multitude of devices using several wired or wireless communication technologies forming a heterogeneous network environment. This environment may include distinct technologies such as Ethernet, Wi-fi, Power Line Communications. To improve the network resource exploitation the IEEE 1905.1 Working Group on Convergent Digital Home Network is designing a technology-independent abstraction layer called Inter-MAC. This layer is in charge of control of the hOME Gigabit Access (OMEGA) network and provides services as well as connectivity to a multitude of devices. In [11, 12] the heterogeneous technologies could converge below the network protocol layer by means of the creation of an intermediate layer: the Inter-MAC. While the combined use of heterogeneous access technologies allows the home network to speeds up to 1 Gps without new wires, the energy consumption in high speed home networks remains an almost unexplored field.

In this paper we show how the combined use of wireless sensor network and OMEGA network can be applied for a mutual advantage. The wireless sensor network can rely on the gigabit network facilities when it is powered up. The gigabit network can be activated and deactivated dynamically relying on an always on and energy efficient wireless sensor network.

The article is organized as follows: in Section 1 the research objectives are clearly identified. In Section 2 the overall research methodology is presented, in terms of architectural design of the proposed solution. In Section 3 we describe the simulation environment used to deploy the designed solution. In Section 4 the simulation environment and the related testbeds are described in detail. In Section 5 the simulation results are analyzed critically to verify the proof of concept. In Section 6 some business benefit in terms of Return Of Investment are highlighted. In Section 7 some conclusions with regard to the obtained results and necessary future work are presented.

2 Objectives

In view of the above the following research objectives have been identified:

1. Define an integrated OMEGA-WSN architecture;
2. Define a Green ICT strategy for home and SOHO scenarios;

3. Define a cost model to determine the economic benefits of using green ICT;
4. Setup a simulation environment to test the proof of concept;
5. Gather the simulation results and perform a critical analysis;
6. If needed, identify potential improvements to be perform in future works.

3 Methodology

The Inter-MAC architecture is presented in [13, 14]. It is divided into data plane, control plane, and management plane. Data plane is responsible for transferring the user/application data packets. It manages the packets arriving at a device, both from the upper layer (network) and the lower MAC/LLC layer. Control plane performs short-term actions in order to manage the data plane behaviour. It is responsible for managing the correspondence between the higher layer application protocol requests and the establishment of new connections or paths to the desired destination with the appropriate QoS requirements. Management plane is concerned with long-term actions which describe the behaviour of the device itself.

To be properly managed, Inter-MAC layer uses a layer 2.5 Inter-MAC protocol. Each OMEGA node, equipped with the Inter-MAC layer functionalities sends and receives proper data and control plane frames. The frame format is shown in Figure 2.

To let the OMEGA network interoperate with a wireless sensor network for a synergic cooperation aiming to save energy, a twofold integration is needed. First of all each energy-consuming OMEGA node must be coupled to a wireless sensor node. Consequently the topology of an integrated OMEGA-WSN network is depicted in Figure 3.

The integration must be applied also in the protocol stack as shown in Figure 4, where a ZigBee protocol stack has been used. Thus the Inter-MAC control and management planes must communicate to perform an intelligent energy save and a rational use of the OMEGA network facilities.

More specifically each OMEGA node can communicate to the sensor node its operational status. The following mean operative states have been defined: (i) Transmission/Reception, (ii) Bridging, and (iii) Idle. In the first case the node is actively participating to provide QoS-aware applications to an end user acting as a sender or as a receiver of the flow. When the node is acting as a network bridge, there is the possibility to deactivate the unused network interfaces. When the node is in idle, there is the possibility to switch

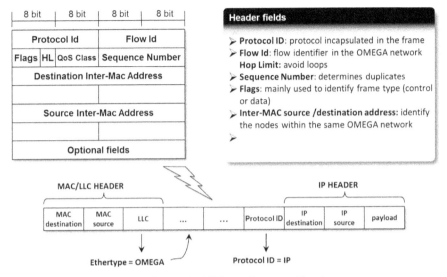

Figure 2 Inter-MAC frame format and header.

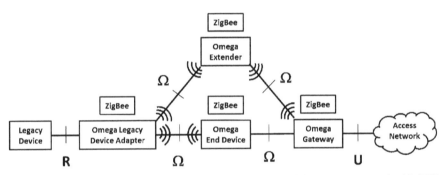

Figure 3 Integrated OMEGA/WSN network: the OMEGA links are represented with "Ω", the last-mile connection is represented with letter "U", the connection between legacy devices and the OMEGA network is represented with "R".

off the whole node in a deep sleep mode. In the last two cases it is possible to save energy, depowering parts of the OMEGA communication systems or the whole node.

As discussed in [15], whenever a new flow must be setup from a source OMEGA node A and a destination OMEGA node B, a broadcast (or unicast) path request control frame is sent at Inter-MAC level, to start up the reactive (or proactive) path selection. The path request control frame flows through the

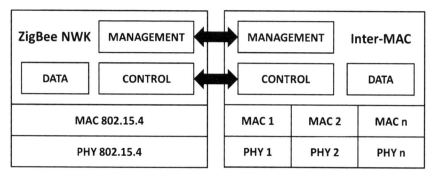

Figure 4 Integrated protocol stack.

OMEGA network from the source node to the destination node to activate the most appropriate path selection algorithm.

In case of an integrated OMEGA+WSN network, the above described message sequence must be adapted to cope with the necessity to intelligently activate the idled or partially operating OMEGA nodes. Whenever a source OMEGA node A needs to setup a new flow towards the destination OMEGA node B, the path request control frame is sent to the Wireless Sensor (WS) node A. The WS node A is in charge to send the broadcast path request over the sensor network that will be intercepted by the WSN node B associated to the destination OMEGA node B. Thus the WSN acts as a dependable control plane, where low data rate control packets can flow even when the OMEGA network is shut down. While the OMEGA nodes or the OMEGA node's network interfaces can be deactivate, the WSN is always on and, due to the low data rate required to properly work, consume a very limited quantity of energy.

When an intermediate WSN node receives a broadcast path request, it activates the OMEGA node and all its interfaces if deactivated, retransmits the broadcast packet (to reach even nodes that are out of range from the source node) and sends an acknowledge packet back to the source WSN node. This awakening phase is needed by the source OMEGA node A to ensure that all the OMEGA nodes are activated when it performs the QoS-aware path selection algorithm to discover the best available path from A to B. Once the path selection solution is known, the OMEGA nodes not involved in the new flow can turn back to their previous idled status. The WSN represents a backup control plane for the OMEGA network able to provide both, a reliable low data rate communication channel and an energy aware protocol to activate

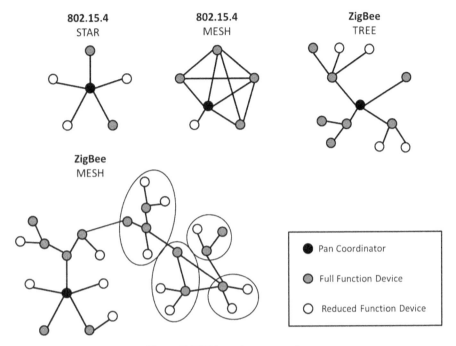

Figure 5 WSN topology examples.

dynamically only the OMEGA nodes needed to provide QoS to the running flows.

Not all the WSNs are feasible for a green ICT scope. As shown in Figure 5, there exist three main WSN topologies: star, tree and mesh. These topologies require an increasing amount of energy.

While in a star topology the always on node is the PAN coordinator, in a tree topology the full function device must perform relatively complex functionalities thus consuming more energy than a simple connected WSN device. In a mesh topology all the nodes are potentially full function devices, thus in the worst case the mesh topology is the less energy efficient. Unfortunately in a indoor environment as a home, or a small office, home office, the presence of walls reduces the communication range between the nodes composing the WSN, thus to ensure the maximum level of reliability and availability of the WSN overlay, a mesh topology (e.g. multicluster ZigBee) is highly recommended.

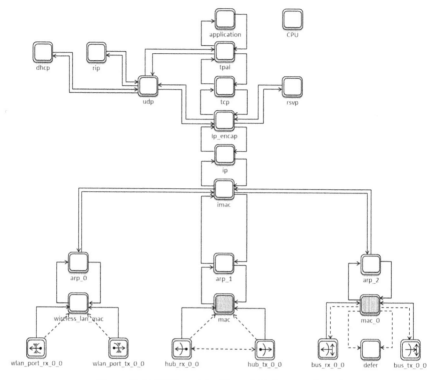

Figure 6 OpNET model of Inter-MAC protocol stack.

4 Technology Description

To demonstrate the validity of the proposed approach, a simulation envir-onment has been setup. The Modeler OPNET 14.5 Educational Version has been used as network simulator for all the tests. It has been preferred against other solutions (NS3, OMNET) for two main reasons. First of all OPNET natively support the technologies needed to perform intensive tests: Ethernet, Wi-Fi and ZigBee. The PLC channel has been approximated using a stat-istical approach described in [15]. On the other hand a particularly accurate OMEGA OpNET model was already available [12,15]. As shown in the Inter-MAC layer has been introduced in the OpNET simulator protocol stack as a new component called imac and located between the layer 3 protocol (IP) and the layer 2 protocols (ARP and MAC). As clearly shown in the Inter-MAC is in charge to interface the IP layer with the heterogeneous underlying technologies: wireless LAN (WLAN), powerline (bus) and Ethernet (hub).

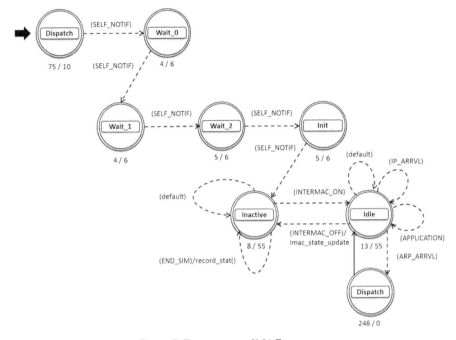

Figure 7 Energy-aware IMAC process.

The OMEGA protocol stack has been modified to cope with the necessity of interfacing with the WSN protocol stack and to manage the operational status of the connected network interfaces and of the whole OMEGA node. This modification has affected mainly the imac finite state machine definition. As shown in Figure 7 a new status has been introduced in the model: inactive. The inactive status means that the OMEGA node is temporary sleeping and needs to be awaken in order to be operative. This status can be modified only by the associated WSN node that, on the contrary, is always running.

The developed WSN node model is depicted in Figure 8. The control_interface process is in charge to manage the communication with the OMEGA node and to simulate the management and control plane interaction with the Inter-MAC layer. As shown in Figure 9 the following main functionalities are provided by the control_interface process:

- APP_CALL – this interrupt is triggered by the OMEGA node control plane. When a new path setup procedure is needed, the OMEGA node invoke the broadcast functionality. The WSN node sends a broadcast wake-up packet over the sensor network. Consequently all the WSN

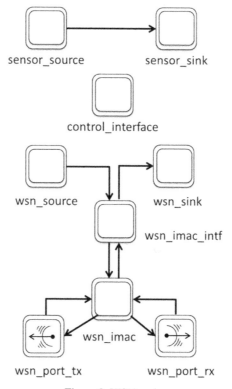

Figure 8 WSN node.

nodes activate the relative OMEGA nodes. Each OMEGA node switch from the inactive status to an idle status. Once the whole OMEGA network is active, the Inter-MAC layer of the source OMEGA node sends over the OMEGA network a Path request packet to trigger the distributed path selection algorithms.

- BROADCAST_RX – this interrupt is triggered when a WSN node intercept a broadcast path request packet. If the relative OMEGA node is inactive an interrupt to the imac process is sent to wake up the OMEGA node or to activate all its network interfaces.
- IMAC_STATE_UPDATE – it is sent by the imac process to update the WSN node with the actual status of the OMEGA node.

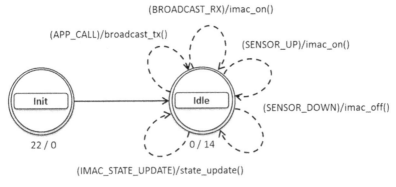

Figure 9 Control-interface process.

5 Developments

The simulation framework has been used to implement different usage scenarios: home network, Small Office Home Office (SOHO) network and Small Enterprise (SE) network. A typical home network is supposed to have less than 10 connected devices. A typical SOHO network is supposed to have up to 50 connected devices, while a SE network may have up to 100 connected devices. Several topologies have been used in the OpNET simulator to generate the most reasonable OMEGA network configurations.

In order to assess the energy saving due to the combined use of OMEGA and WSN networks, the following assumption have been done on the basis of literature and state of the art search (see [17–20] for more details):

- each OMEGA interface (Wi-Fi, Ethernet, Homeplug) has an average energy consumption of 1.5 W;
- each WSN interface has an energy consumption of 0.25 W;
- an average KWh cost of €0.25;
- an average WSN node cost of €4;
- an average OMEGA node energy consumption of 8 W.

Intensive tests have been carried out for the different scenarios. For each scenario multiple tests have been performed to obtain average results. In each test the overall energy consumption has been evaluated applying three different energy saving strategies:

1. No energy saving – the OMEGA network is operative 100% of the time and no WSN is acting to save energy;

2. Partial energy saving – the WSN can solely deactivate the idled interfaces, but not the whole OMEGA node, which is always operative;
3. Maximum energy saving – the WSN can deactivate the whole OMEGA
node when it is in an idle status.

In particular the results have been analyzed in terms of differential benefit obtained applying strategy 2 and 3 against strategy 1. Thus the results represent
the real energy and cost saving associated to the proposed solution.

6 Results

As depicted in Figure 10, the more the OMEGA network is used during a
24 hours duty day, the less the energy saving strategies are effective. Nevertheless a more aggressive energy saving strategy can guarantee a result three
times better than a less aggressive strategy.

The adoption of a maximum energy saving strategy has its own draw-
backs. While an OMEGA node needs less than 1 second to power up and
activate a single network interface, it takes from 20 up to 30 seconds to turn
on the whole OMEGA node and to become fully operative. Thus the best
energy saving strategy must be leveraged with the expected reactive time.
Since a unique applicable solution does not exist, a proper policy must be
decided dynamically or statically to adopt the most appropriate energy saving
strategy.

The efficiency of the proposed strategies can be estimated in terms of
relative energy saving. As shown in Figure 10, having as reference energy
consumption the values associated to the "No energy saving" strategy, and
considering an average network daily use ranging from 12 to 4 hours, the
"Partial energy saving" shows an average efficiency ranging from 13 up to
27%, while the "Maximum energy saving" strategy ranges from 37 up to
75%.

7 Business Benefits

Integrating a wireless sensor network in the OMEGA network incurs an additional cost in terms of acquiring the sensor network and of energy spent
to supply the sensor network. But this initial additional cost can be paid off
from the profit gained by the energy saved in using the OMEGA network.
Considering the above described scenarios, assuming an average use of 4

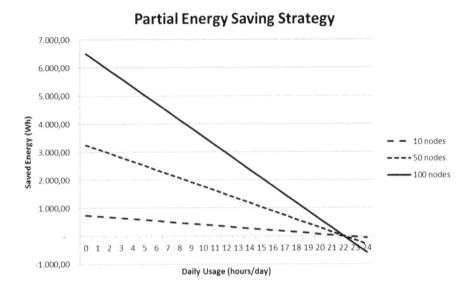

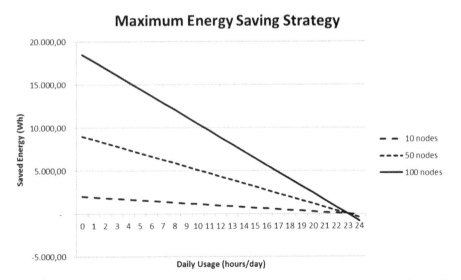

Figure 10 The top graph represents the partial energy saving strategy assuming that each OMEGA node is equipped with two interfaces; the bottom graph represents the maximum energy saving strategy.

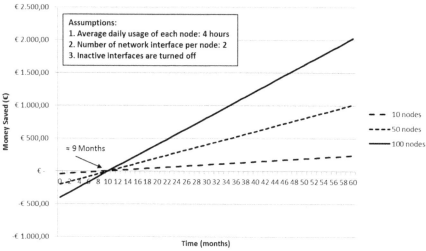

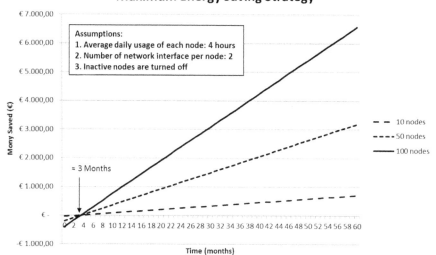

Figure 11 Cost saving results.

hours per day of the OMEGA network and an average of two interfaces for each node, some business benefits can be clearly quantified.

If the strategy adopted is to switch off only the interfaces of a device in idle state than the additional cost is paid off in a period of 9 months for all cases. The average life of the wireless sensor network is estimated to be approximately 5 years. So in this period the benefits are more effective for the scenario with 100 nodes. This fact is depicted in the top graph of Figure 11.

On the other hand, if the energy saving strategy is to totally switch off the inactive nodes the pay off period is reduced significantly to 3 months. In this case even the benefits for the smallest scenario with 10 nodes are substantial and should not be underestimated.

8 Conclusions

In this paper we considered the problem of adopting green ICT technologies in future home networks. We proposed and evaluated an energy saving mechanism by integrating a wireless sensor network with the OMEGA home network. Our strategy dynamically activates and deactivates the gigabit OMEGA network, by means of an always on and energy efficient wireless sensor network. Simulation results show that this mechanism brings substantial long-term benefits due to the energy saved in the overall network, in different usage scenarios.

As a future goal, a better integration of the two networks can be achieved not only in terms of energy saving but also in terms of data plane in order to obtain a mutual benefit. On the one hand, the wireless sensor network can transmit the control messages by using the OMEGA data plane when the nodes are active, and on the other hand the OMEGA nodes can use the wireless sensor network as signalling plane when their interfaces are powered off.

References

[1] International Labour Organization, G20 Statistical update – EU: Heterogeneous shocks and responses across countries, p. 2, April 2009.
[2] A Public-Private Partnership (PPP) for the Future Internet, p. 11, April 2009.
[3] Postnote ICT and CO2 emissions, No. 319, December 2008.
[4] Simon Forge. Powering down: Remedies for unsustainable ICT. *Foresight*, 9(4):3–21, 2007.
[5] Rich Lechner. An inefficient truth. Global Action Plan, IBM, 28 August 2008.

[6] Phil Mckenna. Can we stop the internet destroying our planet? *New Scientist*, 2637, 3 January 2008.

[7] Santad. Visual basic software tool for FTTH network management system. *International Journal of Computer Science and Network Security*, 9(2), February 2009.

[8] M.T. Riaz, J.M. Gutierrez, and J.M. Pedersen. Strategies for the next generation green ICT infrastructure. *Applied Sciences in Biomedical and Communication Technologies*, 2009.

[9] W. Vereecken, W. Van Heddeghem, D. Colle, M. Pickavet, and P. Demeester. Overall ICT footprint and green communication technologies. In *2010 4th International Symposium*, Belgium Communications, Control and Signal Processing (ISCCSP), 2010.

[10] P. Yi Zhang Chowdhury, M. Tornatore, and B. Mukherjee, Energy efficiency in telecom optical networks. *Communications Surveys & Tutorials, IEEE*, 12(4), 2010.

[11] V. Suraci, M. Castrucci, G. Oddi, A. Cimmino, and R. Colella, Convergence in home gigabit networks: Implementation of the inter-MAC layer as a pluggable kernel module. In *Proceedings IEEE PIMRC 2010 Services, Applications, and Business – 21st Annual IEEE International Symposium on Personal, Indoor and Mobile Radio Communication*, 2010.

[12] M. Castrucci, G. Oddi, G. Tamea, and V. Suraci. Application QoS management and session control in a heterogeneous home network using inter-MAC layer support. In *Proceedings Future Network & MobileSummit 2010 Conference*, 2010.

[13] J.P. Javaudin, M. Bellec, D. Varoutas, and V. Suraci. OMEGA ICT project: Towards convergent Gigabit Home Networks. In *Proceedings IEEE PIMRC 2008 – Gigabit Home Access Special Session*, 2008.

[14] F. Delli Priscoli, V. Suraci, and M. Castrucci, Inter-MAC: Convergence at MAC layer in home gigabit network. In *Proceedings 17th ICT-Mobile Summit 2008*, Stockholm, Sweden, 10–12 June 2008.

[15] V. Suraci, D. Macone, and G. Oddi. Load balancing strategy in heterogeneous meshed home access network. Gigabit home and in-building networks, Poster Paper. In *Proceedings ICT-Mobile Summit 2009 Conference*, IIMC International Information Management Corporation, 2009.

[16] OMEGA project website, http://www.ict-omega.eu/.

[17] Tzu-Ming Lin, Power consumption issues for WLAN systems, http://mnet.cs.nthu.edu.tw/paper/tmlin/051209.pdf.

[18] Rahul Balani. Energy consumption analysis for bluetooth, WiFi and cellular networks, http://nesl.ee.ucla.edu/fw/documents/reports/2007/PowerAnalysis.pdf,

[19] Cisco, Ethernet power study of Cisco and competitive products. White Paper, http://www.cisco.com/en/US/prod/collateral/switches/ps5718/ps7077/white_paper_c11-470808.pdf.

[20] Homeplug powerline alliance, HomePlug green PHY specification. White Paper, http://www.homeplug.org/tech/whitepapers/HomePlug_Green_PHY_whitepaper_100614.pdf.

[21] R. Kumar and L. Mieritz. Conceptualizing green IT and data center power and cooling issues. Gartner Research Paper, 2007.

Biography

Vincenzo Suraci was born on November 7, 1978, in Rome, Italy. He graduated in Computer Engineering with 110/110 cum laude in October 2004 at the university of Rome 'Sapienza'. In April 2008 he pursued a Ph.D. in Systems Engineering in the department of Computer Systems Science of University of Rome 'Sapienza'. Currently he is researcher at the university 'e-Campus'.

His main research interest is to develop and to adapt advanced control and operational research theories (reinforcement learning, column generation, hybrid automata, discrete event systems) to solve challenging and emerging engineering problems: connection admission control, access technologies selection in multihoming and inter-home scenarios, semantic service discovery and composition, context-awareness, embedded systems security and dependability, critical infrastructure protection, convergence of heterogeneous networks, quality of experience and quality of service regulation, green ICT.

He has a wide experience in the field of applied research. From year 2005 to 2006 he managed the IMAGES project, an integrated project within the CELTIC research programme. From year 2004 to 2008 he managed the DIADALOS I and DAIDALOS II IP projects within the FP6 EU IST research programme. In 2007 he joined P2P-Next, an IP project within the FP7 EU ICT research programme. From year 2008 to 2011 he managed the OMEGA and MICIE IP projects within the FP7 EU ICT research programme. From 2011 he is managing the Future Internet Core Platform research project: FI-WARE.

Online Manuscript Submission

The link for submission is: www.riverpublishers.com/journal

Authors and reviewers can easily set up an account and log in to submit or review papers.

Submission formats for manuscripts: LaTeX, Word, WordPerfect, RTF, TXT.
Submission formats for figures: EPS, TIFF, GIF, JPEG, PPT and Postscript.

LaTeX

For submission in LaTeX, River Publishers has developed a River stylefile, which can be downloaded from http://riverpublishers.com/river_publishers/authors.php

Guidelines for Manuscripts

Please use the Authors' Guidelines for the preparation of manuscripts, which can be downloaded from http://riverpublishers.com/river_publishers/authors.php

In case of difficulties while submitting or other inquiries, please get in touch with us by clicking CONTACT on the journal's site or sending an e-mail to: info@riverpublishers.com

www.ingramcontent.com/pod-product-compliance
Lightning Source LLC
LaVergne TN
LVHW012332060326
832902LV00011B/1853